Raising a Child with Complex PTSD

What Parents Need to Know to Support, Connect, and Heal Their Traumatized Child

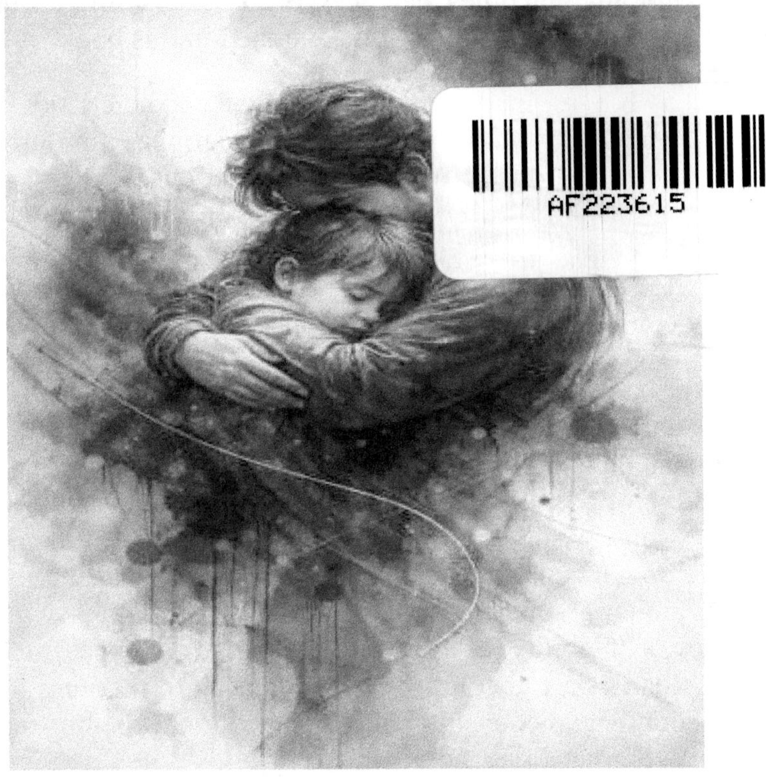

Janet Zufan Rose

Table of Contents

Preface

The sticker chart is not going to work.

Neither is the time-out chair, the lost-privilege consequence, the calm-down jar from Pinterest, or the behavior contract the school counselor printed from a template. You have tried them. You have tried all of them. You have read the mainstream parenting books, attended the workshops, followed the Instagram accounts, and implemented the strategies with consistency, patience, and genuine effort. And your child still rages for 45 minutes over a change in the dinner plan. Still goes blank in the middle of a conversation and stares through you as though you are not there. Still tells you they hate you with a ferocity that takes your breath away, then climbs into your lap 20 minutes later as though nothing happened. Still performs beautifully at school and falls apart the moment they walk through your front door.

The advice has not failed because you applied it wrong. It has failed because it was designed for a different kind of child. Specifically, it was designed for a child whose brain developed inside a safe enough caregiving environment, a child whose nervous system learned, in the first years of life, that adults are predictable, that needs will be met, and that the world is more safe than dangerous. The strategies assume a foundation that your child does not have. And until someone explains why that foundation is missing and what to build in its place, every parenting tool in the world will bounce off your child like instructions written in the wrong language.

Complex Post-Traumatic Stress Disorder in children is not a rare clinical footnote. It is a condition affecting millions of children worldwide who have endured prolonged, repeated exposure to abuse, neglect, domestic violence, or institutional deprivation during the developmental window when the brain is most vulnerable to disruption. The World Health Organization recognized CPTSD as a distinct diagnosis in the ICD-11 in 2018, differentiating it from single-event PTSD by three additional features: chronic emotional dysregulation, a pervasive negative self-concept, and persistent difficulty in relationships. In children, these features do not present as tidy diagnostic criteria. They present as meltdowns that last an hour. As food hoarded under mattresses in a house with a full refrigerator. As a teenager who earns straight A's through anxious compliance and then shatters at home because there is nowhere left to perform. As behaviors that are consistently misread as defiance, manipulation, or poor discipline by the very systems designed to help.

The parents and caregivers raising these children, through adoption, foster care, kinship placement, or reunification, are parenting without a manual that addresses their actual reality. Mainstream parenting advice was built for children whose nervous systems developed in safety. Traditional discipline depends on a child who can connect cause to effect, who trusts that the adult means well, and who is motivated by approval. For a child with CPTSD, every one of those preconditions may be absent. The result is a parent who loves their child fiercely and feels like they are failing every day, surrounded by advice that does not apply, professionals who may not understand the diagnosis, and a community that judges the child's behavior and the parent's response without seeing either one clearly.

The neuroscience offers a different story. The brain that was shaped by trauma can be reshaped by safety, attunement, and consistent caregiving. Neuroplasticity, the brain's capacity to form new pathways in response to new experiences, is especially strong in developing children. Research on children placed in stable, responsive environments after early adversity shows measurable recovery in emotional regulation, cognitive functioning, and attachment patterns. Healing is not a metaphor. It is a neurological process, and the primary instrument of that process is the relationship between the child and the adults who choose to stay.

But that relationship cannot do its work if the adults do not understand what they are dealing with. A parent who interprets dissociation as defiance will respond with consequences that deepen the child's shutdown. A caregiver who reads a fawn response as cooperation will miss the terror underneath the compliance. A family that relies on sticker charts and time-outs will watch those tools fail repeatedly and conclude that the child, not the approach, is the problem.

The book in your hands was written to close that gap. It translates the clinical research on complex developmental trauma into language that belongs in the living room, not the lecture hall. It covers the neuroscience of CPTSD in children, the failure of traditional behavioral approaches and what to use instead, evidence-based therapeutic modalities and how to access them, crisis management and safety planning, school advocacy and legal protections, the impact on siblings and partnerships and extended family, caregiver mental health and sustainability, and the long-term trajectory of healing from childhood through emerging adulthood. Every chapter includes composite case studies drawn from common family experiences, practical tools that can be implemented immediately, and references to peer-reviewed research for those who want to go deeper.

The chapters are designed to be read sequentially for a complete understanding or accessed individually when a specific crisis or question demands immediate guidance. Appendices include printable worksheets, screening checklists, advocacy letter templates, a glossary of key terms, and a curated directory of organizations and resources.

No book can replace a qualified trauma therapist. No book can undo what has already been done to a child. What a book can do is help the adults in that child's life understand what they are seeing, respond in ways that heal rather than harm, and sustain themselves through a process that is longer and harder than anyone warned them it would be. The research says the prognosis improves dramatically when the caregiving environment changes.

The caregiving environment is you. This is where the work begins.

Janet Zufan Rose
Researcher and Author

Part One: Understanding the Storm

— What Complex PTSD Is and Why Your Child Behaves This Way

Chapter 1.0 Not What You Expected

Parenting books tend to follow a familiar pattern. They describe a problem, offer a technique, and promise that consistency will pay off. And for many families, that pattern works well enough. But you may be reading this because none of that has worked for your family. The techniques fell flat. The consistency made things worse. The advice your pediatrician gave, the tips from well meaning relatives, the consequences your child's school recommended, all of it seemed to bounce off your child like rain off glass.

This chapter is about naming that experience honestly. If you are raising a child who has lived through repeated, overwhelming stress (and if their behavior leaves you confused, exhausted, and sometimes frightened) this book was written for the space you're standing in right now.

When Morning Feels Like a Minefield

Consider Elowen (name changed), a foster mother of two years. She described a typical Tuesday morning this way. Her seven year old daughter woke up screaming at 5:14 a.m. from the same nightmare she'd had three times that week. By the time Elowen reached her room, the child had pulled all the sheets off the bed and was crouched in the corner, eyes wide, breathing hard, not recognizing Elowen's face. It took 20 minutes of sitting on the floor, speaking quietly, before the girl came back to the present.

Breakfast was a negotiation. The cereal was wrong. The spoon was wrong. The chair was wrong. Elowen knew from experience that what looked like pickiness was actually her daughter's nervous system scanning for anything unfamiliar, anything that might signal danger. By 7:30 a.m., there had been a meltdown over socks (the seam felt wrong), a refusal to brush teeth (the toothpaste burned last time at her old house), and a 10 minute freeze in the hallway where her daughter simply stopped moving and stared at the wall.

Elowen got her daughter to school on time. She smiled at the teacher, buckled her seatbelt, drove to the parking lot of a grocery store, and cried for 15 minutes before going to work.

That was a good morning.

If any part of Elowen's story sounds familiar to you, this book is here to help you understand what is happening, why it is happening, and what you can do about it (without losing yourself in the process).

The Silence Around This

One of the hardest parts of raising a child with Complex PTSD is how isolating it can feel. There are support groups for parents of children with ADHD. There are well known books about parenting autistic children. There are school programs, social media communities, and pediatric specialists for a wide range of childhood conditions. But when your child's struggles stem from repeated traumatic experiences, especially relational ones like abuse, neglect, or exposure to violence, the resources become thin. The conversation becomes quieter.

Part of this is clinical. Complex PTSD (CPTSD) is still a relatively new concept in mainstream mental health. It was only formally included in the World Health Organization's International Classification of Diseases (ICD-11) in 2018, and it is still absent from the DSM-5, the diagnostic manual most commonly used in the United States (World Health Organization, 2018). That means many clinicians have not been trained to recognize it, especially in children.

Part of it is social. Parenting a traumatized child often involves situations that other families simply cannot relate to. A child who hoards food under their bed. A child who rages for 90 minutes and then goes completely blank. A child who tells their teacher that you hurt them, even though you didn't, because that is the only relational pattern their brain knows. These are not experiences you can easily share at a school pickup line.

Consider Bramwell (name changed), a kinship caregiver who took in his niece after she was removed from a home with domestic violence. He described feeling "like I was parenting a child no one had written the manual for." He tried rewards. He tried structure. He tried gentle parenting. He tried strict boundaries. Nothing was consistently effective, because the techniques were designed for children whose nervous systems had a reliable baseline of safety. His niece did not have that baseline.

If you recognize yourself in Bramwell's experience, you are carrying something heavy. And the fact that you are still here, still reading, still looking for answers, says something about your commitment to this child.

Why Everything You Tried Fell Short

Before we go any further, something needs to be said plainly. If the parenting strategies you've tried so far have not worked, that does not mean you are a bad parent. It means the strategies were built for a different kind of child.

Most parenting advice assumes a child who has a baseline sense of safety. A child whose nervous system trusts that the adults around them are predictable, that the world follows certain rules, and that feelings can be expressed without catastrophic results. Children with CPTSD do not have that baseline. Their brains were shaped by environments where the rules changed without warning, where the people who were supposed to be safe were also the source of harm, and where emotional expression could bring punishment instead of comfort.

When you apply traditional behavioral strategies (sticker charts, time outs, privilege removal, logical consequences) to a child whose nervous system is wired for survival, the strategies often backfire. A time out that is meant to encourage reflection can feel, to a traumatized child, like abandonment. A consequence designed to teach accountability can be experienced as proof that this home, too, is a place where adults use power to control.

We will go much deeper into this in Chapter 5.0. For now, the point is simply this: if you've been trying everything and nothing has worked, the problem is likely not your effort. The problem is a mismatch between the tool and the situation.

Consider Crispin (name changed), a foster father who described spending six months implementing a carefully designed behavior chart with his 10 year old foster son. The child earned stickers for completing morning routines and lost privileges for aggression. After six months, the aggression had increased, and the child had begun hiding the behavior chart in the trash. "I thought I was doing everything right," Crispin said. "I read all the books. I was consistent. And it was getting worse." What Crispin did not yet know was that his son's aggression was a trauma response, not a behavioral choice. And the interventions designed for behavioral choices were unintentionally telling the child that his pain was a problem to be managed with stickers.

What This Book Will Do

This book will give you a working understanding of Complex PTSD as it shows up in children. Not in clinical jargon, but in plain language tied to the behaviors you actually see. It will explain why your child's brain and body respond the way they do. It will give you practical, evidence based approaches for daily parenting, crisis moments, school advocacy, and your own emotional health.

Each chapter is built around real problems that parents in your situation face. You will find case studies (with changed names) drawn from common patterns in clinical and caregiving literature. You will find specific language you can use, questions you can bring to your child's providers, and tools you can put into practice the same week you read them.

This is not a book that tells you to love harder. Love matters. But love without understanding can accidentally cause harm, and this book is here to close that gap between what your heart wants to do and what your child's brain actually needs.

What This Book Won't Do

This book is not a replacement for therapy. It is a companion to therapy, for your child and for you. It does not diagnose your child. It does not prescribe medication. It does not promise that if you follow every step, everything will be fine by next Tuesday.

Healing from developmental trauma is slow, nonlinear, and deeply individual. What this book can do is make the road more understandable, less lonely, and more grounded in what the research actually shows.

If your child is currently in crisis or you are concerned about immediate safety, please contact a crisis professional before continuing with this book. The resources in Appendix C include crisis hotlines and emergency contacts.

Reading This Your Way

You can read this book from front to back. The chapters build on each other, starting with understanding (Part One), moving through practical parenting shifts (Part Two), addressing therapy and treatment (Part Three), covering crisis and systems (Part Four), and ending with your own wellbeing (Part Five).

But you can also use it as a reference. If your child is in the middle of a meltdown right now, go to Chapter 12.0. If you have an IEP meeting next week, go to Chapter 13.0. If you are trying to figure out if your child's diagnosis is right, Chapter 4.0 was written for that specific question. If your marriage is suffering under the weight of this, Chapter 14.0 addresses that directly. If you need to understand why your child dissociates, Chapter 3.0 covers the brain science in plain terms.

Each chapter stands on its own while connecting to the others. Cross references will point you to related material. And every chapter ends with a summary and references so you can go deeper on anything that matters to you.

A note on pace. This is a long book that covers difficult material. You do not need to absorb it all at once. Some chapters may bring up feelings that catch you off guard. That is normal. Set the book down when you need to. Come back when you're ready. It will be here.

Words Matter

Throughout this book, you will see the phrase "child with CPTSD" or "child who has experienced complex trauma." These are deliberate choices. Your child is not "a CPTSD kid." They are not defined by what happened to them. They are a child, first and always, who is carrying the weight of experiences that should never have happened.

You will also notice that this book does not assume your family looks a certain way. You may be a biological parent, a foster parent, an adoptive parent, a grandparent, an aunt, an uncle, or a family friend who stepped in when no one else could. The word "parent" in this book means you: the person who shows up every day for this child. Your relationship to this child is defined by your presence, not by biology or legal paperwork.

Similarly, this book does not assume your child's trauma came from one type of experience. Neglect, abuse, medical trauma, family instability, community violence, and institutional care all produce complex trauma responses. Whatever your child's story, the principles in this book apply.

And this book will never tell you that loving your child is enough on its own. Love is the starting point. But love paired with understanding becomes something much more effective. That pairing is what we're building here.

Putting It Together

This chapter set the stage. You now know that the experience of raising a child with Complex PTSD is distinct from other parenting challenges, that the clinical world is still catching up to what families like yours have known for years, and that this book is built to serve you as a practical, compassionate guide.

In Chapter 2.0, we begin with the question most parents ask first: what is Complex PTSD, exactly, and how is it different from everything else my child has been diagnosed with?

Chapter 2.0 Complex PTSD Explained

When parents first hear the term "Complex PTSD," the reaction is often a mixture of relief and confusion. Relief, because finally there is a name for what they have been watching their child go through. Confusion, because this name does not show up on most diagnostic reports, and it may not be something their child's doctor has ever mentioned.

This chapter explains what Complex PTSD actually is, how it differs from regular PTSD, why it matters for your child, and what it looks like at different ages. By the end, you will have a clear picture of the condition that may be driving your child's most confusing behaviors.

What CPTSD Actually Means

Complex Post Traumatic Stress Disorder (CPTSD) is a condition that develops after prolonged, repeated exposure to traumatic events, particularly when those events happen during childhood and involve the people who were supposed to provide care and safety (World Health Organization, 2018). The word "complex" is not just a clinical label. It describes the layered, tangled nature of the damage. This is not one bad thing that happened once. This is an accumulation of harmful experiences, often stretching over months or years, woven into the fabric of a child's daily life.

The World Health Organization included CPTSD in the ICD-11, its international diagnostic system, in 2018. The ICD-11 describes CPTSD as having all the features of PTSD (re-experiencing the trauma, avoidance of reminders, and a persistent sense of threat) plus three additional clusters of symptoms. Those three clusters are what make CPTSD different from standard

PTSD, and they are what most parents recognize immediately in their children (Cloitre et al., 2013).

Three Pillars of CPTSD

The first cluster is **emotional dysregulation**. This means the child has severe difficulty managing their emotional responses. They may swing from rage to numbness in seconds. They may have reactions that seem wildly out of proportion to the situation. A spilled glass of milk triggers a 45 minute screaming episode. A compliment causes tears. A transition from one activity to another brings on a shutdown where the child stares blankly and cannot respond. These reactions are not choices. They are the product of a nervous system that learned, through repeated danger, to stay in emergency mode (van der Kolk, 2014).

The second cluster is **negative self concept**. Children with CPTSD often carry a deep, persistent belief that they are bad, worthless, damaged, or fundamentally different from other people. This is not low self esteem in the way that a shy child might feel unsure of themselves. It is a core belief, built during the years when the child's sense of self was forming, that they deserved what happened to them. They may say things like "I'm stupid," "Nobody wants me," or "I ruin everything." These statements are not attention seeking. They reflect what the child genuinely believes about themselves, because the adults who were supposed to teach them their worth either failed to do so or actively taught them the opposite (Herman, 2015).

The third cluster is **disturbed relationships**. Children with CPTSD struggle with connection. They may desperately want closeness but push people away the moment they feel vulnerable. They may trust strangers too quickly or trust no one at all. They may test your commitment by behaving in ways designed (often unconsciously) to make you reject them, because rejection is the outcome their brain expects. They may also become extremely compliant and "good," not because they feel safe, but because they learned that being invisible was the safest way to survive (Ford & Courtois, 2020).

Consider Aldwyn (name changed), a nine year old adopted from foster care at age five. His parents described him as "two different kids." At school, he was quiet, cooperative, and eager to please. Teachers described him as a model student. At home, he screamed, threw things, refused food, and told his parents he hated them. His parents were baffled. But this pattern makes sense through the lens of CPTSD. At school, Aldwyn was in "fawn" mode, performing compliance to avoid perceived danger. At home, where he felt just safe enough to stop performing, the pain and dysregulation poured out.

How CPTSD Differs From PTSD

Standard PTSD typically develops after a single traumatic event or a time limited series of events: a car accident, a natural disaster, a violent assault. The person re-experiences that specific event through flashbacks, nightmares, and intrusive memories. They avoid reminders of that event. They feel on edge and hypervigilant (American Psychiatric Association, 2013).

CPTSD is different in its origins and in its effects. It develops not from a single event, but from a pattern of events, often occurring during the critical years of brain development. And because the trauma is usually relational (caused by or related to caregivers), it affects not just how the child responds to danger, but how they see themselves, how they connect with others, and how they regulate every emotional experience they have (Cloitre et al., 2013).

Think of it this way. PTSD is like a wound that needs to heal. CPTSD is like growing up in an environment where the wound never had a chance to form a scab, because the source of the injury was also the source of care.

Why the Diagnosis Might Not Say CPTSD

If CPTSD has been an official diagnosis since 2018, why doesn't your child's paperwork reflect it? The answer lies in which diagnostic system your providers use. In the United States, most clinicians use the DSM-5, published by the American Psychiatric Association. The DSM-5 does not include CPTSD as a separate diagnosis. It includes PTSD with a broader set of symptoms than previous editions, but it does not recognize the distinct cluster of self concept, emotional regulation, and relational disturbances that define CPTSD (American Psychiatric Association, 2013).

The ICD-11, used widely in Europe and recognized by the World Health Organization, does include CPTSD. This means that depending on where you live and which system your child's clinician uses, the same child could receive very different diagnostic labels for the same set of symptoms.

This is not just an academic distinction. It has real consequences. Without a recognized diagnostic code, insurance companies may not cover treatments specifically designed for complex trauma. Schools may not understand how to accommodate a child whose struggles go beyond standard PTSD. And parents may spend years chasing a correct diagnosis while their child accumulates labels that don't capture what is actually going on.

Developmental Trauma Disorder

Researchers Bessel van der Kolk and Julian Ford proposed a diagnosis called **Developmental Trauma Disorder** (DTD) specifically for children whose complex trauma began early in life and affected their development. DTD captures what CPTSD looks like in a growing child: disrupted attachment, problems with emotional and physical regulation, behavioral difficulties, cognitive impairments, and a distorted sense of self (van der Kolk, 2005).

DTD was proposed for inclusion in the DSM-5, but was not accepted, partly due to concerns about the research base at the time. The clinical community continues to advocate for it, and many trauma specialists use the concept in their practice even without a formal diagnostic code (Ford & Courtois, 2020).

For parents, the takeaway is this: if your child's presentation does not seem to fit neatly into any single DSM-5 diagnosis, it may be because the diagnosis that best describes their experience is not yet in the book their clinician is required to use.

What Leads to CPTSD in Children

CPTSD does not come from one type of experience. It can develop from chronic physical, emotional, or sexual abuse. It can develop from persistent neglect, both physical and emotional. It can come from living in a household with domestic violence, from repeated medical trauma (painful procedures, extended hospitalizations, especially in infancy), from prolonged separation from primary caregivers, from institutional care in orphanages or group homes with inadequate staffing, from community violence over extended periods, or from having a caregiver with untreated severe mental illness or addiction.

The common thread is duration, repetition, and the involvement of someone the child depends on for safety. A single frightening event can cause PTSD. But when the fear is built into the daily fabric of a child's life, especially during the years when their brain is forming its basic templates for safety, relationships, and self worth, the result is CPTSD (Spinazzola et al., 2018).

Consider Crispin (name changed), a 12 year old whose early years were spent with a parent who alternated between warmth and unpredictable rage, depending on substance use. Crispin did not experience one traumatic event. He experienced thousands of moments in which the person he loved most became the person he feared most. His brain learned that love and danger come from the same source. By the time he entered a stable foster home at age eight, that learning was wired deeply into his responses.

How It Looks at Different Ages

In toddlers and preschoolers (ages two to five), CPTSD often presents as regression. A child who was toilet trained begins having accidents. A child who was speaking begins to withdraw into silence. Sleep disturbances, night terrors, clinginess, extreme tantrums, and sensory sensitivities are common. At this age, the child lacks the language to describe what they feel, so the body and behavior carry the message (Perry & Szalavitz, 2006).

In school age children (ages six to 12), CPTSD may show up as aggression, lying, stealing, difficulty with peers, academic struggles, controlling behavior, and what looks like deliberate defiance. The child may have trouble concentrating (which is often mistaken for ADHD), difficulty reading social cues (which may be mistaken for autism), and explosive reactions to small frustrations (which may be labeled as ODD). We will address the misdiagnosis issue in depth in Chapter 4.0.

In teenagers (ages 13 to 18), CPTSD can present as risk taking, substance use, self harm, dissociation, problems with authority, difficulty maintaining friendships or romantic relationships, and either a highly controlled exterior masking inner chaos or an outwardly chaotic life that mirrors the internal state. Teens with CPTSD are at higher risk for running away, school dropout, involvement with the justice system, and early sexual activity, not because they are "bad kids," but because these behaviors represent the survival strategies their brains have learned (Cook et al., 2005).

Consider Dunstan (name changed), a 15 year old whose mother brought him to therapy after he was caught stealing from a classmate. His therapist initially explored conduct issues. But when the family history revealed years of witnessing violence between his parents before their separation, the therapist shifted focus. Dunstan was not stealing because he lacked morals. He was operating from a nervous system that had never learned to feel safe enough to trust that his needs would be met. Taking what he needed was a survival behavior, not a character flaw.

What This Means For You

Understanding CPTSD changes the way you see your child. It shifts the question from "What is wrong with them?" to "What happened to them, and how did their brain adapt to survive it?" That shift is not just compassionate. It is clinically accurate. And it opens the door to approaches that actually work, which is where we are headed in the chapters to come.

In Chapter 3.0, we look inside your child's brain to understand exactly why their nervous system behaves the way it does. That knowledge will become the foundation for every practical strategy in this book.

Chapter 3.0 The Brain Under Siege

If you have ever watched your child go from calm to explosive in a matter of seconds, if you have seen them freeze in the middle of a conversation and go somewhere you cannot reach, if you have noticed that their body seems to react before their mind even has a chance to think, then you have already seen the effects of trauma on the developing brain.

This chapter explains what is happening inside your child's brain and body when they behave in ways that confuse or frighten you. This is not academic information for its own sake. Every practical strategy in this book rests on the science in this chapter. When you understand why your child's nervous system does what it does, you stop taking the behavior personally and start responding in ways that actually help.

Two Brains in One

Your child essentially has two operating systems running at the same time. The first is the **survival brain**, sometimes called the lower brain or the limbic system. This part of the brain is ancient, fast, and automatic. It is responsible for detecting danger, triggering the stress response, and keeping the child alive. It does not think. It does not reason. It reacts (Perry & Szalavitz, 2006).

The second is the **thinking brain**, centered in the prefrontal cortex. This part of the brain handles reasoning, planning, impulse control, empathy, cause and effect thinking, and emotional regulation. It is the part that allows a child to pause before acting, consider consequences, and make a thoughtful choice (Siegel, 2012).

Here is what matters for your child. In a healthy, safe environment, the thinking brain gradually develops the ability to manage the survival brain. A toddler who screams when frustrated is using their survival brain. By age eight or nine, most children can name the feeling, take a breath, and choose a different response. That's the thinking brain coming online.

But in a child with CPTSD, repeated trauma has kept the survival brain in a near constant state of activation. The alarm system has been on so long that it has become the default setting. And because trauma often occurs during the critical years when the prefrontal cortex is developing, that development can be disrupted. The thinking brain has not had the chance to build the connections it needs to manage the survival brain effectively (van der Kolk, 2014).

This is why your child can seem perfectly capable of making good decisions sometimes, and then act as though they have no capacity for reason at all in the next moment. When the survival brain takes over, the thinking brain goes offline. Your child is not choosing to be difficult. They are literally operating from a different part of their brain.

The Alarm That Won't Turn Off

The **amygdala** is a small, almond shaped structure deep in the brain that acts as the body's alarm system. Its job is to scan the environment for threat and trigger the stress response when danger is detected. In a child who has experienced repeated trauma, the amygdala is overactive. It has been trained by experience to see danger everywhere, even in situations that are objectively safe (LeDoux, 2015).

This is why your child may react to a raised voice (even a happy, excited one) as though they are in danger. This is why a change in routine, which feels minor to you, can send them into a spiral. The amygdala does not distinguish between a real threat and something that resembles a threat. It fires first and asks questions later. Or rather, it fires first and the thinking brain (if it comes back online) asks questions later.

Consider Fenwick (name changed), an eight year old who had been in his adoptive home for three years. His father described an evening when the family was watching a movie together. A character in the film raised his hand suddenly, and Fenwick dove off the couch and crawled under the coffee table, covering his head. There was no danger. But Fenwick's amygdala did not know that. It recognized the motion of a hand going up. It fired. And Fenwick's body responded before his conscious mind had any say in the matter.

Stress Hormones on Overdrive

When the amygdala signals danger, the body's stress response system kicks in. The **HPA axis** (hypothalamic pituitary adrenal axis) releases cortisol and adrenaline, preparing the body to fight or flee. Heart rate increases. Muscles tense. Digestion slows. The immune system shifts into emergency mode (Gunnar & Quevedo, 2007).

In a healthy stress response, the danger passes, cortisol levels drop, and the body returns to baseline. But in children who have lived with chronic threat, the HPA axis can become dysregulated. Cortisol may stay elevated for long periods, or it may become blunted (the body stops producing normal amounts because it has been flooded for so long). Both patterns create problems. Chronically elevated cortisol can impair memory, weaken the immune system, and interfere with growth. Blunted cortisol can leave a child appearing flat, disconnected, or unable to respond to normal social cues (Gunnar & Quevedo, 2007).

This is one reason why children with CPTSD often have physical complaints: headaches, stomachaches, fatigue, frequent illness, and sensory sensitivities. Their bodies are carrying the burden of a stress response system that never fully turns off.

How the Nervous System Responds

Researcher Stephen Porges developed what is called **polyvagal theory**, which describes three states the nervous system can operate in. Understanding these states will help you recognize what your child is experiencing in real time (Porges, 2011).

The first state is called **ventral vagal**, or the "safe and social" state. In this state, the child feels calm, connected, and able to engage with others. Their face is expressive, their voice has normal tone and rhythm, and they can make eye contact comfortably. This is the state where learning, play, and relationship building happen.

The second state is **sympathetic activation**, or the "fight or flight" state. In this state, the child's body has mobilized for action. Heart rate is up. Muscles are tense. They may become aggressive (fight), try to run or escape (flight), or become restless and unable to sit still. This is the state that teachers often see as "behavior problems." The child is not misbehaving. They are mobilized for survival.

The third state is **dorsal vagal**, or the "shutdown" state. This is what happens when the nervous system decides that fighting and fleeing are both impossible. The body conserves energy by going still. Heart rate drops. The child may appear spaced out, glazed, unresponsive, or emotionally flat. Some children describe it as "going away" or "being somewhere else." This is dissociation, and it is one of the most misunderstood trauma responses in children (Porges, 2011).

Some researchers and clinicians also describe a **fawn** response, where the child responds to perceived threat by becoming excessively agreeable, compliant, and focused on pleasing the other person. This is the child who is "too good," who never makes waves, who anticipates adult needs and meets them before being asked. It can look like maturity, but it is actually a survival strategy rooted in the belief that safety depends on keeping others happy (Walker, 2013).

Consider Godric (name changed), a 10 year old whose mother described him as having "three settings." In Setting 1, he was warm, funny, and engaged (ventral vagal). In Setting 2, he was reactive, angry, and physical (sympathetic activation). In Setting 3, he sat on the couch and stared at nothing, and no amount of calling his name brought him back for 10 to 15 minutes (dorsal vagal shutdown). His mother said, "It's like he leaves the room without moving his body." She was exactly right. Godric's nervous system was cycling through these states because it had learned, through years of unpredictable caregiving, that no state was permanently safe.

The Window of Tolerance

Psychiatrist Daniel Siegel introduced the concept of the **window of tolerance** to describe the zone of arousal in which a person can function well. Inside the window, a child can think, feel, process, and respond to the world. Above the window, they are in hyperarousal (anxious, reactive, aggressive). Below the window, they are in hypoarousal (shut down, numb, dissociated) (Siegel, 2012).

For most children, the window of tolerance is reasonably wide. They can handle a certain amount of stress, frustration, and change without flipping into either extreme. For children with CPTSD, the window of tolerance is narrow. Sometimes it is barely a crack. This means that very small provocations (a loud noise, a surprise, a "no") can push them out of their window and into a state where their thinking brain goes offline and their survival brain takes the wheel.

Now, here's what gives this chapter its weight. The window of tolerance can be widened. Through safe, attuned relationships, through co-regulation with a calm adult, and through appropriate therapeutic support, children can gradually expand their capacity to stay in the zone where they can think and connect. We will discuss exactly how to support this process in Chapters 6.0 and 7.0.

Memory and Triggers

Trauma is stored differently in the brain than ordinary experience. Most memories are processed through the hippocampus, which organizes them with a time stamp and context. You remember what happened, when it happened, and that it is over. These are called **explicit memories** (Siegel, 2012).

Trauma memories, especially those formed in early childhood, are often stored as **implicit memories**: fragments of sensation, emotion, and body response without a narrative or time stamp. The child does not remember the event as a story. They re-experience it as a feeling, a smell, a sound, or a bodily sensation, and they may have no idea why. The body responds as though the danger is happening right now, because the brain has not filed the memory into the "past" category (van der Kolk, 2014).

This is why triggers can seem irrational. A particular tone of voice. A certain kind of lighting. The smell of a particular food. The feel of a specific fabric. The child's amygdala recognizes the sensory fragment, sounds the alarm, and the stress response fires before the thinking brain has any chance to say, "Wait, that was then. This is now."

Consider Hadrian (name changed), a six year old who screamed and ran every time his foster father started cooking with onions. It took months before the family learned that Hadrian's biological father used to cook with onions before episodes of violence. Hadrian could not articulate this. He did not have a conscious memory of the connection. But his body remembered.

When the Body Speaks

Children with CPTSD frequently experience physical symptoms that seem unrelated to trauma: chronic stomachaches, headaches, muscle tension, fatigue, difficulty sleeping, bedwetting, appetite problems, and heightened sensitivity to sensory input (noise, touch, texture, light). These are not imaginary complaints. They are the physical expression of a nervous system that has been running in emergency mode for months or years (van der Kolk, 2014).

Some children also show sensory processing difficulties that look similar to sensory processing disorder. They may be overwhelmed by certain textures, unable to tolerate tags in clothing, or intensely reactive to sounds. When these symptoms arise in the context of trauma history, they may reflect the body's hypervigilant scanning for threat rather than a standalone sensory condition.

The Brain Can Change

And now the part that matters most. The human brain, especially a young one, is capable of remarkable change. The scientific term for this is **neuroplasticity**, and it means that the neural pathways formed by trauma can be reshaped through new experiences (Perry & Szalavitz, 2006).

Healing does not mean erasing the past. It means building new pathways alongside the old ones. It means giving your child enough repeated experiences of safety, attunement, and co-regulation that their brain begins to update its predictions. "Maybe this adult is safe." "Maybe I can feel this feeling without falling apart." "Maybe the danger is over."

This does not happen fast. And it does not happen through words alone. It happens through relationship, through consistency, and through the steady, patient presence of a caregiver who understands what the child's brain needs and provides it, day after day, even when the child pushes back.

That is what the rest of this book is about.

Your Next Steps

Your child's brain has been shaped by experiences that kept it in survival mode. The alarm system is overactive. The thinking brain is still developing. The stress hormones may be dysregulated. And the memories of trauma are stored in fragments that can be triggered by things that seem harmless.

None of this is your child's fault. And none of it is permanent. The brain that was wired for danger can be gradually rewired for safety. You are a central part of that process. The next chapters will show you how.

Chapter 4.0 The Diagnostic Maze

If you have been to three different specialists and received four different diagnoses for the same child, you are not losing your mind. You are experiencing one of the most frustrating realities of raising a child with Complex PTSD: the condition looks like almost everything else.

This chapter explains why CPTSD is frequently misdiagnosed, how its symptoms overlap with other common childhood diagnoses, and what you can do to advocate for a more accurate understanding of your child. You will also find a practical checklist of questions to bring to your child's next evaluation.

The Great Imitator

Clinicians and researchers who specialize in developmental trauma have called CPTSD "the great imitator" because its symptoms map onto the criteria for so many other diagnoses. A child with CPTSD may have difficulty concentrating (looks like ADHD). They may have explosive emotional reactions (looks like bipolar disorder). They may refuse to follow directions (looks like ODD). They may struggle with social cues and sensory input (looks like autism). They may show extreme emotional instability (looks like early borderline personality traits). And they may have attachment difficulties (looks like RAD) (van der Kolk, 2005).

The problem is not that clinicians are careless. The problem is that the diagnostic tools they use (primarily the DSM-5) do not include CPTSD as a standalone diagnosis. So they are working with the categories they have. And the categories they have were designed to capture symptoms, not causes. Two children can meet the criteria for ADHD based on identical behavioral checklists, yet one has a neurodevelopmental condition and the other has a traumatized nervous system mimicking the same presentation (Szymanski et al., 2011).

This distinction is not academic. It changes treatment entirely. A child with true ADHD may respond well to stimulant medication and behavioral interventions. A child whose concentration problems stem from chronic hyperarousal may be made worse by those same treatments, because the underlying problem is an overactive stress response, not a dopamine deficit.

CPTSD and ADHD

The overlap between CPTSD and ADHD is one of the most common sources of misdiagnosis in children. Both conditions can produce difficulty paying attention, restlessness, impulsivity, and trouble completing tasks. But the mechanism is different (Szymanski et al., 2011).

In ADHD, attentional difficulties come from neurodevelopmental differences in executive functioning. They are present across settings and contexts, typically from early childhood, and they do not fluctuate dramatically based on emotional state.

In CPTSD, the child's attentional difficulties come from hypervigilance. Their brain is scanning for danger instead of focusing on the teacher. They are distracted not by boredom or a wandering mind, but by the constant low level alarm running in their nervous system. Their restlessness comes from a mobilized stress response, not from excess energy. And their impulsivity often spikes in situations that trigger a trauma memory, then drops in settings where they feel safe.

Questions that help distinguish the two: Did the attention problems begin before or after the traumatic experience? Do they improve in safe, predictable environments? Are they accompanied by hypervigilance (scanning for exits, watching adults' faces, flinching at sudden sounds)? Does the child dissociate (go blank, seem to leave the room mentally) as well as lose focus?

Consider Ivor (name changed), an 11 year old who had been diagnosed with ADHD at age seven and prescribed stimulant medication. The medication helped somewhat with focus at school, but his meltdowns at home intensified. His new therapist, trained in trauma assessment, conducted a thorough developmental history and discovered that Ivor's first four years had been spent in a home with severe domestic violence. Re-evaluation suggested that his inattention was driven by chronic hyperarousal. When his treatment shifted to trauma focused therapy and his parents learned co-regulation strategies (which we cover in Chapter 7.0), his symptoms improved more than they ever had on medication alone.

Ivor's story is not unusual. A study published in the *Journal of Infant, Child, and Adolescent Psychotherapy* found that trauma and ADHD share more overlapping symptoms than distinguishing ones, making the risk of misdiagnosis and missed diagnosis very high (Szymanski et al., 2011).

CPTSD and ODD

Oppositional Defiant Disorder is characterized by a pattern of angry, irritable mood, argumentative behavior, and defiance or vindictiveness. Many children with CPTSD meet these criteria. But the behavior has a different origin (Ford & Courtois, 2020).

In ODD (as traditionally conceptualized), the defiance is seen as a behavioral pattern that can be addressed with consistent limit setting, consequences, and behavioral modification. In CPTSD, what looks like defiance is often a survival response. The child learned that compliance can be dangerous ("If I do what adults tell me, bad things happen"). Their "no" is not a power struggle. It is a protective barrier between themselves and a world that has proven itself unsafe.

When a child with CPTSD is treated exclusively with behavioral interventions designed for ODD (point systems, escalating consequences, loss of privileges), the interventions often fail because they do not address the underlying fear. Worse, they can escalate the child's distress by confirming their belief that adults use power to control and harm.

CPTSD and Bipolar Disorder

Bipolar disorder in children is characterized by episodes of mania (elevated or irritable mood, rapid speech, decreased need for sleep, grandiosity) alternating with episodes of depression. The emotional swings of CPTSD can look similar, particularly the rapid shifts between intense anger and flatness or withdrawal (Cloitre et al., 2013).

The difference lies in the pattern and the trigger. In bipolar disorder, mood episodes tend to last days or weeks and are not consistently tied to environmental triggers. In CPTSD, emotional shifts are typically triggered by something (even if the trigger is not immediately obvious) and can happen moment to moment. A child with CPTSD may go from rage to collapse in 10 minutes, not because of a mood cycle, but because a sensory trigger activated their stress response and the collapse is their nervous system shutting down after the surge.

Misdiagnosis as bipolar disorder can lead to medication with mood stabilizers or antipsychotics that do not address the underlying trauma and may carry side effects the child does not need to bear.

CPTSD and Autism

The overlap between CPTSD and autism spectrum conditions is increasingly recognized in clinical literature. Both can involve difficulty with social interaction, sensory sensitivities, rigid or repetitive behaviors, difficulty with transitions, and challenges reading social cues (Kerns et al., 2015).

In autism, these features are neurodevelopmental. They are present from birth (though they may not be recognized until later), they are consistent across settings, and they are part of the child's neurological wiring.

In CPTSD, social withdrawal may come from mistrust rather than difficulty with social cognition. Sensory sensitivities may reflect a hypervigilant nervous system (as we discussed in Chapter 3.0) rather than a sensory processing difference. Rigidity around routines may be an attempt to create predictability in a world that felt chaotic, rather than an innate preference for sameness. And some children with CPTSD have learned to suppress emotional expression to the point where they appear flat, which can be mistaken for the reduced emotional display sometimes associated with autism.

It is also possible for a child to be both autistic and have CPTSD. In those cases, the autism came first and the trauma may have been compounded by the child's vulnerability. Sorting out which symptoms belong to which condition requires careful, thorough assessment by a clinician experienced with both.

CPTSD and RAD

Reactive Attachment Disorder (RAD) is sometimes used interchangeably with CPTSD in casual conversation, but they are different. RAD is a specific attachment disorder, most often seen in children who experienced severe neglect or institutionalization in early life. It is characterized by a consistent pattern of inhibited, emotionally withdrawn behavior toward caregivers (American Psychiatric Association, 2013).

A child can have CPTSD without having RAD. CPTSD affects emotional regulation, self concept, and relationships broadly, while RAD specifically describes the absence of healthy attachment behavior. Many children with CPTSD show disordered attachment (sometimes insecure, sometimes disorganized), but they may still seek proximity to caregivers, which would not be consistent with a RAD diagnosis.

Collecting Diagnoses

Consider Jory (name changed), a 13 year old whose file included the following diagnoses accumulated over six years: ADHD, ODD, generalized anxiety disorder, intermittent explosive disorder, and rule out bipolar disorder. Five labels. None of them included the word "trauma."

Jory's mother described feeling like she was "collecting diagnoses the way other people collect stamps." Each specialist saw one slice of Jory's presentation, named it according to the tools they had, and moved on. No one stepped back to ask the unifying question: what happened to this child, and how did their brain adapt?

This experience, sometimes called "diagnostic overshadowing," is common among children with complex trauma histories. The symptom picture is so broad that it generates multiple labels, each one addressing a piece of the puzzle while missing the pattern that ties them together (Spinazzola et al., 2018).

If your child has multiple diagnoses and none of them seem to capture the full picture, it may be time to seek an evaluation from a clinician who specializes in developmental trauma. The questions below can help guide that conversation.

Questions for Your Child's Provider

Bring this list to your child's next evaluation or treatment review:

- Has my child's trauma history been formally assessed as part of the diagnostic process?
- Are you familiar with Complex PTSD as defined in the ICD-11, and with the concept of Developmental Trauma Disorder?
- Could any of my child's symptoms be explained by chronic hyperarousal, dissociation, or disrupted attachment rather than the current diagnoses?

- Are we treating the root cause or managing surface symptoms?
- Have we considered that my child's attention difficulties might stem from hypervigilance rather than ADHD?
- Would a trauma focused assessment change the treatment plan?
- What training have you had in recognizing complex trauma presentations in children?
- If I sought a second opinion from a trauma specialist, would you support that?

You are not being difficult by asking these questions. You are being a thorough advocate for your child.

When It Truly Is Both

Not every child with a trauma history has been misdiagnosed. Some children genuinely have CPTSD and another condition. A child can be autistic and traumatized. A child can have ADHD and CPTSD. A child can have a mood disorder and complex trauma. These are not mutually exclusive.

The key is ensuring that trauma is part of the clinical picture, not erased by it. If your child has ADHD and CPTSD, they need treatment for both. Stimulant medication alone will not resolve the hypervigilance. Trauma therapy alone will not address the neurodevelopmental component. A good treatment plan holds all the pieces.

Consider Kenrick (name changed), a nine year old who was diagnosed with ADHD at age five, before his adoption. After adoption, his parents noticed symptoms that ADHD did not explain: hoarding food, flinching at raised voices, night terrors, and intense distress around transitions. A subsequent trauma assessment identified CPTSD alongside the existing ADHD diagnosis. His treatment was expanded to include both stimulant medication (for the neurodevelopmental ADHD) and trauma focused therapy (for the CPTSD). Both pieces were necessary.

The Bottom Line

Getting the right diagnosis matters because it determines the right treatment. If your child's CPTSD symptoms are labeled as ADHD, they will receive ADHD treatment. If they are labeled as ODD, they will receive behavioral modification. If they are labeled as bipolar, they will receive mood stabilizers. None of those treatments address the underlying trauma.

You do not need to become your child's diagnostician. But you can be their advocate. Ask the questions. Bring the history. Request a trauma informed assessment. And remember that a child can have more than one condition at the same time.

In Chapter 5.0, we move from understanding to action. Now that you know what your child is dealing with and why traditional approaches often miss the mark, we look at what to do differently.

Part Two: Rethinking Everything

Why Traditional Parenting Doesn't Work and
What Does

Chapter 5.0 Why Sticker Charts Don't Stick

Traditional parenting rests on a set of assumptions that most people never question, because for most children, those assumptions hold true. The child feels safe. The child trusts the adults in their life. The child can connect cause to effect. The child believes that following rules leads to good outcomes and breaking rules leads to bad ones. From these assumptions flow the techniques that fill mainstream parenting books: reward charts, time outs, logical consequences, and escalating privilege loss.

This chapter explains why those techniques consistently fail with children who have Complex PTSD, and why continuing to use them can actually deepen the harm. This is not about blaming you for trying them. You were using the tools you were given. The problem is that those tools were designed for a different situation.

The Hidden Assumptions

Every parenting strategy carries invisible assumptions about the child it was designed for. Sticker charts assume the child can delay gratification, that they believe the promised reward will actually arrive, and that they feel motivated by adult approval. Time outs assume the child can self regulate when alone, that brief separation feels uncomfortable but not threatening, and that the child will use the quiet time to reflect. Logical consequences assume the child understands cause and effect, that they connect today's behavior with tomorrow's loss of privilege, and that they believe the system is fair (Purvis et al., 2013).

For a child with CPTSD, every one of these assumptions may be wrong.

A child who grew up with unkept promises does not believe the sticker chart reward will arrive. A child whose early caregivers disappeared or became dangerous does not experience time out as a brief pause; they experience it as abandonment. A child whose world was governed by chaos and unpredictability does not connect today's behavior to tomorrow's consequence, because in their formative experience, consequences were random and unrelated to their actions (Perry & Szalavitz, 2006).

This is not a failure of intelligence or willfulness. It is a neurological reality. As we discussed in Chapter 3.0, the thinking brain (prefrontal cortex) is the part that handles cause and effect reasoning, impulse control, and future oriented thinking. In children with CPTSD, that part of the brain is frequently offline, overridden by a survival brain that is focused on one question: Am I safe right now?

When Consequences Backfire

Consider Larkin (name changed), a 10 year old in an adoptive family who had been through three foster placements before finding permanency. His parents implemented a behavior management system recommended by a well meaning therapist: green, yellow, and red cards displayed on the refrigerator. Green meant a good day. Yellow meant warnings. Red meant loss of screen time and early bedtime.

Within two weeks, Larkin began deliberately escalating to red every morning. His parents were confused. Why would a child choose to lose privileges? But Larkin was not making a strategic choice. He was doing what his nervous system demanded. The card system introduced uncertainty (Will I stay green? When will I fail?) that felt intolerable. By pushing to red immediately, Larkin eliminated the uncertainty. The bad thing had already happened. He could stop waiting for it.

His parents described feeling like they were "punishing him into worse behavior." They were exactly right. The consequence system was not reducing the unwanted behavior. It was increasing Larkin's anxiety, which increased the dysregulation, which increased the behavior the system was supposed to address.

This pattern is well documented in trauma literature. Consequences that depend on the child's ability to self regulate fail when the child's self regulation capacity is impaired by chronic stress. The child cannot meet the expectation, so they fail. The failure triggers shame. The shame activates the stress response. And the stress response produces more of the behavior the adult was trying to stop (Hughes & Baylin, 2012).

Why Punishment Fails the Traumatized Brain

Punishment, whether it takes the form of spanking, yelling, privilege removal, or enforced isolation, relies on the child experiencing discomfort and connecting that discomfort to their behavior. The theory is that the child will want to avoid the discomfort in the future, and will therefore change their behavior.

For a child with CPTSD, punishment activates the trauma response. A raised voice does not register as "I should make a different choice next time." It registers as danger. Isolation does not register as "time to think about what I did." It registers as the familiar experience of being left alone when things get bad. Even the removal of a privilege does not register the way it's intended, because for many traumatized children, expecting good things to be taken away is baseline. It is what they already believe will happen (van der Kolk, 2014).

Punishment also reinforces the negative self concept that is already a core feature of CPTSD (as described in Chapter 2.0). A child who already believes they are bad, worthless, or unlovable hears punishment as confirmation. "See? I knew I was terrible. Now you know it too." The punishment does not motivate change. It deepens despair.

Consider Merrick (name changed), an eight year old whose grandmother was raising him after his removal from a home with chronic neglect. When Merrick hit another child at school, the school's response was a three day suspension. His grandmother described his reaction: "He came home and said, 'They don't want me there either.' He wasn't sorry about hitting. He was just adding another place to the list of places that had gotten rid of him."

The hitting was a problem that needed addressing. But the suspension addressed it in a way that made Merrick's core wound worse. He did not learn to manage his anger. He learned that this place, like every other place, would push him out when he was too much.

The Myth of Willful Defiance

"He knows better." "She does it on purpose." "He can behave when he wants to, so this is a choice."

These are some of the most common things said about children with CPTSD, and they are some of the most damaging. The reasoning goes like this: if the child behaves well in one setting (such as school) but falls apart in another (such as home), then the problem must be willpower, not ability. If they can hold it together for six hours, the argument goes, then the meltdown at home is a choice.

This reasoning misunderstands how the nervous system works. As we discussed in Chapter 3.0, a child with CPTSD may spend the school day in fawn mode, performing compliance in an environment that feels unsafe. That performance is not evidence of self regulation. It is evidence of survival strategy. By the time they get home (the one place where they feel just safe enough to stop performing) the nervous system collapses. The meltdown is not defiance. It is the release of hours of accumulated stress that had nowhere to go (Bomber, 2007).

Think of it like holding your breath underwater. A person might hold their breath for 90 seconds. When they surface, they gasp. You would not say, "Well, you were fine for 90 seconds, so the gasping must be a choice." The gasping is the body's automatic response to an unsustainable state. That is what is happening when your child melts down after a day of "good behavior."

Consider Oswin (name changed), a 14 year old whose teachers consistently reported that he was "a pleasure to have in class." His foster parents could not reconcile this with the child who came home and screamed, slammed doors, and once put his fist through a bedroom wall. The discrepancy was used against them. A school counselor suggested that the behavior at home was "attention seeking" and that the parents needed to "stop walking on eggshells." But Oswin's therapist, trained in complex trauma, explained the pattern: Oswin was using every ounce of his regulatory capacity to hold it together at school. When he walked through the front door, the capacity was spent. The behavior at home was not a choice. It was the cost of the performance.

The Bad Kid Story

When a child with CPTSD is repeatedly punished for behavior they cannot control, a story begins to take shape in their mind. Not a story they consciously write, but one that forms from the pattern of their experience. The story goes something like this: I am the kind of person who gets in trouble. I am the kind of person who makes people angry. I am the kind of person who cannot get things right.

This story is what clinicians call a negative self narrative, and it becomes self reinforcing. The child acts out because their nervous system is dysregulated. They get punished. The punishment confirms that they are bad. The shame of being bad increases their dysregulation. The increased dysregulation produces more acting out. And the cycle continues (Hughes & Baylin, 2012).

Every consequence that is delivered without first addressing the underlying fear adds a brick to this wall of negative self concept. Every "What is wrong with you?" or "We've talked about this a hundred times" or "I'm so disappointed" tells the child that the adults in their life see the same worthless person the child already believes themselves to be.

This does not mean you cannot have expectations. It does not mean you let the child do whatever they want. It means the way you frame expectations and respond to unmet expectations matters enormously for a child whose self concept is already fragile. We will get into specific strategies for this in Chapters 6.0 and 7.0.

Grieving the Parenting You Imagined

There is one more thing that needs to be named in this chapter, and it is not about your child. It is about you.

Most parents enter parenthood (whether biological, adoptive, or foster) with an image of what it will look like. There will be hard moments, of course, but the techniques will work. The rewards will motivate. The boundaries will hold. The child will learn. The parenting books will be relevant.

When you discover that none of this applies to your child, something is lost. The parenting experience you imagined is not the one you are living. And that loss deserves to be named as grief, because that is what it is.

You may grieve the relationship you expected to have with this child. You may grieve the ease you see in other families. You may grieve the version of yourself that was confident and competent, before this experience made you feel like you were failing every day. You may even grieve the child you thought you were getting, which can come with its own layer of guilt.

None of this grief means you love your child less. It means you are human, and you are adjusting to a reality that is harder than anything you prepared for. Acknowledging that grief is not weakness. It is the beginning of being honest about what you need, which is something we address directly in Chapter 16.0.

Where This Leads

If traditional parenting techniques don't work for your child, what does? The answer begins with a concept called felt safety, which is the subject of the next chapter. Felt safety is the foundation that was supposed to be built during your child's earliest years but wasn't. Everything that follows in this book (every strategy, every script, every intervention) rests on that foundation.

In Chapter 6.0, we start building it.

Chapter 6.0 Felt Safety First

There is a difference between being safe and feeling safe. Your child may live in a stable home with a full refrigerator, a warm bed, and adults who would never harm them. They may be, by every objective measure, safe. But their nervous system does not know that yet.

This chapter introduces the concept of felt safety, which is the internal, body level experience of being safe enough to let your guard down. For children with CPTSD, building felt safety is not one strategy among many. It is the strategy. Everything else (emotional regulation, behavior change, relationship building, academic progress) depends on it.

Neurological Safety vs. Physical Safety

When we talk about safety for most children, we mean the absence of physical danger. The doors are locked. The smoke detectors work. The adults are responsible. And for children whose nervous systems developed normally, physical safety and felt safety are closely aligned. They feel safe because they are safe.

For a child with CPTSD, the connection between physical safety and felt safety has been severed. Their brain learned its safety templates during a time when the environment was dangerous, when the people who were supposed to protect them were also the source of harm. Those templates do not update automatically when the environment changes. The child's thinking brain may know, intellectually, that this home is different. But the survival brain is not convinced (Baylin & Hughes, 2016).

This is why your child may flinch when you reach for a hug. Why they may refuse food from you but eat freely at a friend's house. Why they may test your limits with behavior that seems designed to provoke rejection. The survival brain is running old software. It is interpreting your home through the lens of the environment it was trained in. And it will keep doing so until it accumulates enough new evidence to rewrite its predictions.

Building felt safety means providing that new evidence, consistently, patiently, and through the body as much as through words.

The PACE Model

One of the most widely used frameworks for building felt safety with traumatized children is the **PACE model**, developed by clinical psychologist Dan Hughes. PACE stands for Playfulness, Acceptance, Curiosity, and Empathy (Hughes, 2009).

Playfulness does not mean being silly when your child is in distress. It means bringing lightness, warmth, and gentle humor into the relationship during calm moments. Playfulness signals safety to the nervous system because play is a ventral vagal activity (as described in Chapter 3.0). When a caregiver is playful, the child's brain registers: this person is relaxed, which means there is no danger. Playfulness can be as simple as a funny voice during morning routines, a spontaneous dance in the kitchen, or a lighthearted comment when things go slightly wrong ("Oh no, the toast is extra crunchy today. I think the toaster is showing off.").

Acceptance means communicating that you accept the child's inner experience, even when you cannot accept their behavior. A child who screams "I hate you" is expressing pain. Acceptance sounds like: "You're really angry right now. That feeling makes sense." It does not mean agreeing with the child or allowing harmful behavior. It means separating the emotion (which is always valid) from the action (which may need to be redirected).

Curiosity replaces judgment. Instead of "Why did you do that?" (which a traumatized child hears as an accusation), curiosity sounds like "I wonder what was happening for you right before that." Curiosity communicates that you are trying to understand, not trying to punish. It invites the child into a collaborative process of making sense of their experience, rather than placing them on the defensive.

Empathy is the capacity to sit with your child's pain without trying to fix it, minimize it, or rush past it. Empathy sounds like "That sounds really hard" or "I can see this is a lot for you right now." It does not require you to have experienced what your child experienced. It requires you to be willing to feel alongside them, even when what they feel is uncomfortable.

Consider Quinlan (name changed), a foster father who had been parenting his seven year old foster son for eight months. The child refused to make eye contact, spoke in monosyllables, and ate every meal as though someone might take the plate away. Quinlan described feeling "like I was living with a ghost." A therapist introduced PACE, and Quinlan began making small shifts. During meals, he stopped commenting on the child's eating speed and instead talked about his own day in a warm, casual tone (playfulness). When the child flinched at a loud sound, Quinlan said, "That was a big noise. Makes sense you didn't like it" (acceptance and empathy). When the child shoved his plate off the table, Quinlan said, "Huh. I wonder if something about dinner felt wrong" (curiosity). The changes were not dramatic. But after three months, the child began occasionally looking at Quinlan while he talked. After five months, the child asked him a question at dinner for the first time. Felt safety was building, one interaction at a time.

Predictability and Routine

For a child whose early life was chaotic, predictability is medicine. When they can anticipate what comes next, the survival brain has one less thing to scan for. The thinking brain gets a small window to come online. Over time, repeated predictability begins to teach the nervous system that this environment follows rules that hold (Purvis et al., 2013).

Building predictability does not mean rigidity. It means creating a framework the child can count on. Morning routines that follow the same sequence. Meals at roughly the same time. Bedtime rituals that do not change without warning. Transitions that are announced before they happen ("In 10 minutes, we're going to leave for school. In 5 minutes, we'll put on shoes.").

Surprises are particularly activating for children with CPTSD. Even pleasant surprises (a spontaneous trip to the park, an unexpected gift) can trigger the alarm system, because "unexpected" and "dangerous" are linked in the child's implicit memory. This does not mean you can never be spontaneous. It means that in the early stages of building felt safety, predictability should be the default.

When routines must change, give as much advance notice as possible. Use concrete, visual supports (a picture schedule, a written list, a whiteboard with the day's plan). And name the change directly: "Today is going to be a little different. Here's what's going to happen."

Consider Elowen (name changed), the foster mother we met in Chapter 1.0. After learning about felt safety, she created a visual morning schedule with pictures for each step: wake up, use the bathroom, get dressed, eat breakfast, brush teeth, put on shoes. She posted it on the wall at her daughter's eye level. The meltdowns did not disappear. But they shifted. Instead of every step being a potential crisis, the child began checking the schedule between steps. She still struggled with transitions, but the predictability gave her something to hold onto. "The schedule became her anchor," Elowen said. "She trusted the wall more than she trusted me. And that was okay. The wall was a start."

The Sensory Environment

Children with CPTSD often have heightened or dysregulated sensory processing. Loud noises, bright lights, certain textures, strong smells, or unexpected physical contact can all activate the alarm system. Creating a sensory aware environment is not about making your house a therapy clinic. It is about reducing the number of triggers that compete for your child's attention throughout the day (Warner et al., 2013).

Practical adjustments include dimming lights in the evening or using warm toned bulbs. Reducing background noise (turning off the television when no one is watching, using a white noise machine for sleep). Offering clothing choices that prioritize comfort over appearance. Being attentive to food textures and temperatures. And building in physical movement throughout the day, because movement helps discharge the energy that accumulates in a mobilized stress response.

Safe Spaces

A safe space is a designated area in your home where your child can go when they feel overwhelmed. It is not time out. It is not punishment. It is a resource the child can choose, and that distinction matters enormously.

A safe space might be a corner of a room with soft blankets, stuffed animals, a weighted lap pad, noise canceling headphones, and a few sensory tools (fidgets, putty, a snow globe). The child can go there when they feel their window of tolerance narrowing (Chapter 3.0), and they can stay as long as they need.

The key is that the safe space is introduced during calm moments, not during crisis. Practice using it together. Let the child help design it. Frame it explicitly: "This is your spot for when feelings get big. It's not because you're in trouble. It's because everyone needs a place to feel safe."

Fifteen Felt Safety Interventions By Age

The following interventions are organized by developmental stage. Choose the ones that fit your child's current functioning level, which may not match their chronological age.

Ages Two to Five

Offer choices between two acceptable options instead of open ended questions ("Do you want the blue cup or the green cup?" instead of "What do you want to drink?"). Narrate daily activities in a calm voice ("Now we're washing hands. The water is warm. We use soap."). Use a transition object (a small toy or fabric) that travels with the child between settings. Maintain a consistent bedtime ritual with the same sequence each night. Sit at the child's physical level during conversations and keep your voice low and slow.

Ages Six to Twelve

Create a visual daily schedule the child can check independently. Offer a "heads up" before any change to routine or expectation. Build in a decompression period after school before any demands are made (20 to 30 minutes of unstructured, low demand time). Teach one simple body based calming strategy (slow breathing, wall push ups, squeezing a stress ball) and practice it during calm moments. Use collaborative problem solving instead of top down directives: "We have a problem. The morning is hard. What could we try together?"

Ages Thirteen to Eighteen

Respect the teen's growing need for autonomy by involving them in decisions about routines and expectations. Offer sensory supports without framing them as childish (weighted blankets, fidgets, music with headphones). Create a texting code or hand signal the teen can use to communicate "I need space" without having to explain in the moment. Make car rides a regular low pressure connection point (sitting side by side instead of face to face reduces threat). Acknowledge their experience without trying to fix it: "That sounds rough. I'm here if you want to talk, and I'm here if you don't."

The Long Game

Building felt safety is not a technique you apply for two weeks and evaluate. It is a way of being with your child that accumulates over months and years. Some days you will see progress. Many days you will wonder if anything is changing. It is.

Consider Aldwyn (name changed), the nine year old we met in Chapter 2.0. Six months after his parents began implementing PACE, predictable routines, and a safe space in his room, his mother described the change this way: "He still has hard days. He still screams sometimes. But last week, after a meltdown, he came to me and said, 'I'm sorry I yelled.' He has never done that before. He has never come back after a rupture. That's new. That's the felt safety working."

Progress with felt safety does not look like the absence of difficult behavior. It looks like shorter recovery times. It looks like the child coming to you after a rupture instead of withdrawing. It looks like a moment of eye contact that was not there six months ago. It looks like trust, building slowly and unevenly, from the inside out.

Bringing It Forward

Felt safety is the soil. Without it, nothing else grows. With it, everything in the chapters ahead becomes possible. In Chapter 7.0, we move from building the foundation to living on it, day by day. You will learn how to use connection as your primary parenting tool, how to set limits with warmth, and exactly what to say in the 10 situations that trip up parents most often.

Chapter 7.0 Connection Before Correction

If Chapter 6.0 built the foundation, this chapter is about what happens every day on top of it. This is the chapter you will return to most often, because it addresses the moments that fill your actual life: the morning when your child refuses to get dressed, the dinner when they throw food, the bedtime when they cling to you and then shove you away, and the car ride home from school when something clearly happened but they won't tell you what.

Traditional parenting says: set the boundary, deliver the consequence, stay consistent. Trauma informed parenting says: connect first. Correct second. And always, always lead with relationship.

Relationship as the Intervention

When clinicians talk about evidence based treatment for childhood CPTSD, they emphasize a concept called "relational repair." The injury happened in relationship (with caregivers who were unavailable, dangerous, or unpredictable). The healing also happens in relationship, with caregivers who are present, safe, and attuned (Hughes & Baylin, 2012).

This means that you, the parent, are not just the person who drives your child to therapy. You are the therapy. Your consistent presence, your steady voice, your willingness to stay in the room when your child pushes you away, these are the active ingredients of healing. Every interaction is an opportunity to teach your child's nervous system something new: that connection is safe, that adults can be trusted, and that being seen does not lead to being harmed.

This does not mean every interaction must be perfect. It means the pattern of your interactions matters more than any single moment.

Co-Regulation

Before a child can learn to regulate their own emotions, they need to borrow your regulation. This is called **co-regulation**, and it is the biological foundation of emotional development (Siegel, 2012).

In typical development, co-regulation begins in infancy. A baby cries, and the caregiver responds with a calm voice, a steady presence, and physical comfort. The baby's nervous system learns to settle in response to the caregiver's settled state. Over thousands of repetitions, the child internalizes this pattern and develops the ability to settle themselves.

For children with CPTSD, those thousands of repetitions either did not happen or happened inconsistently, often interspersed with responses that increased the child's distress rather than calming it. The neural pathways for self regulation were not built. And you cannot build them with instructions. You cannot tell a child to "calm down" and expect it to work, any more than you can tell someone who never learned to swim to "just float."

What you can do is lend your calm. When your child is dysregulated, the most powerful thing you can do is regulate yourself first (which is harder than it sounds, and we will address that in Chapter 16.0). Your calm, steady presence gives their nervous system something to anchor to. Lower your voice. Slow your breathing. Reduce your words. Offer your physical presence without forcing contact. The child's mirror neurons pick up on your state and begin to pattern match. Not instantly. Not every time. But over hundreds of interactions, the template builds.

Consider Bramwell (name changed), the kinship caregiver from Chapter 1.0. He described a turning point in his understanding of co-regulation. His niece was screaming and throwing shoes in the hallway. His instinct was to raise his voice and tell her to stop. Instead, he sat down on the floor, leaned against the wall, and said quietly, "I'm right here. I'm not going anywhere." She screamed for another 10 minutes. Then she threw one more shoe (weakly). Then she sat down next to him. They sat in silence for five minutes. "I didn't fix anything," Bramwell said. "I didn't solve the problem. But she came toward me instead of running away. That had never happened before."

That moment was co-regulation in action. Bramwell's calm body communicated safety. His niece's nervous system, after exhausting its sympathetic activation (the screaming and throwing), detected a safe anchor and moved toward it.

Attunement and Rupture Repair

Attunement means accurately reading your child's emotional state and responding in a way that tells them they have been seen. It does not mean getting it right every time. Even the most attuned parents misread their children. What matters is what happens after the misread.

In healthy development, the cycle of attunement, rupture (missing the child's cue), and repair (coming back and reconnecting) teaches the child that relationships can survive mistakes. The child learns that disconnection is temporary and that the adult will return. For children with CPTSD, this lesson was never learned. In their experience, rupture was permanent, or it was followed by something dangerous.

Repair is therefore one of the most therapeutic things you can do. When you lose your temper (and you will), when you respond with frustration instead of empathy, when you miss the cue and your child feels unseen, come back. Say, "I got that wrong. I was frustrated, and I didn't listen the way I should have. I'm sorry. Can we try again?" (Siegel & Bryson, 2011).

This teaches your child something radical: that adults can make mistakes without becoming dangerous, that anger does not mean abandonment, and that the relationship is stronger than the rupture.

Naming the Feeling, Not the Behavior

When your child throws their dinner plate, the instinct is to name the behavior: "Don't throw things." When they scream that they hate you, the instinct is to address the words: "That's not how we talk."

Trauma informed parenting reverses this. Name the feeling first. Address the behavior second. "You're really angry right now" comes before "and we keep food on the table." "Something is hurting you" comes before "and I need the words to be different."

This sequence matters because the feeling is what's driving the behavior. If you address only the behavior, the feeling stays unresolved and will find another outlet. If you address the feeling first, you give the child the experience of being understood, which in itself begins to de-escalate the stress response (Hughes, 2009).

Time Ins Instead of Time Outs

A time out sends the child away from the relationship at the exact moment they need it most. A **time in** brings the relationship to the child.

A time in might look like sitting with the child in a quiet space. It might mean reducing stimulation (turning off lights, lowering voices, moving to a calmer room). It might involve offering a blanket, a drink of water, or a fidget tool. The message is:

"You're having a hard time, and I'm going to stay with you through it." Not: "Go away until you can behave."

This does not mean the child faces no limits. It means the limits come after the nervous system has settled, when the thinking brain is back online and the child can actually process what you're saying. Delivering a consequence during a meltdown is like trying to teach someone grammar while they're drowning. First you pull them out of the water. Then, later, you talk about grammar.

Setting Limits with Warmth

Some parents worry that trauma informed parenting means having no boundaries. It does not. Children with CPTSD need boundaries. Clear, consistent, predictable boundaries are part of felt safety (Chapter 6.0). What changes is how you deliver and enforce them.

The formula is connection, then limit, then reconnection.

"I can see you're really frustrated (connection). Hitting isn't safe, so I'm going to move the blocks out of reach for now (limit). When you're ready, we can try again together (reconnection)."

"You wanted to keep playing, and it's hard to stop (connection). It's time for bed because your body needs rest (limit). I'll sit with you while you settle in (reconnection)" (Purvis et al., 2013).

The limit is the same as it would be in any parenting approach. What changes is the emotional wrapper around it. The child hears: I see your feeling. I'm holding the boundary. And I'm not leaving.

When Connection Is Rejected

Some children with CPTSD will push you away when you try to connect. They will say, "Leave me alone." They will slam doors.

They will refuse your comfort, your presence, and your help.
This is not evidence that connection does not work. It is evidence
that connection is exactly what they are most afraid of.

For these children, connection was paired with danger. The closer
they got to a caregiver, the more they got hurt. Their brain
learned: connection equals vulnerability, and vulnerability equals
pain. So they reject it preemptively, before it can hurt them again.

Consider Godric (name changed), the 10 year old we met in
Chapter 3.0. When his mother tried to comfort him after a
meltdown, he would scream "Don't touch me!" and hide under
his bed. His mother felt helpless. But his therapist coached her to
stay present without forcing contact. She would sit outside his
bedroom door and say, "I'm right here. I'm not coming in, but I'm
not leaving either." Over time, Godric began leaving his door
cracked open. Then sitting closer to the doorway. Then, one
evening, reaching his hand out and touching her shoe. That was
his way of testing: is this person still here even when I push?

The answer needs to be yes, even when it is painful.

Consider Merrick (name changed), the eight year old from
Chapter 5.0, whose grandmother was raising him. When she first
tried time ins, Merrick would shove her away and yell, "I don't
need you!" She described wanting to cry. But she kept showing
up. She would sit a few feet away, stay quiet, and wait. One
afternoon, after 20 minutes of shoving and yelling, Merrick
stopped. He looked at her. He said, "You're still here." She said,
"I'm still here." He climbed into her lap and fell asleep. He was
testing the one question his entire history had taught him to ask:
will this person stay when I'm at my worst? That afternoon, for
the first time, he got the answer his nervous system needed.

Scripts for Ten Common Flashpoints

Here are specific phrases you can use in the moments that come up most often. These are not magic words. They are templates built on the principle of connection before correction.

When your child says "I hate you": "You're feeling something really big right now. I'm here, even when you're angry at me."

When they refuse to do a transition (get dressed, leave the house, come to dinner): "I can see this switch is hard. Your body isn't ready yet. Let's take a minute, and then we'll do it together."

When they hit, kick, or throw things: "I'm going to keep us both safe. I can see how upset you are. Let's find another way to get that feeling out."

When they lie about something obvious: "I think something about telling the truth feels scary right now. I'm not mad. I just want to understand what happened."

When they refuse food: "Your stomach gets to decide. The food will be here if you change your mind."

When they melt down at bedtime: "Nighttime can feel big and hard. I'm going to stay close. You don't have to be okay right now."

When they regress (baby talk, clinginess, bedwetting): "Your body is telling me it needs some extra comfort right now. That's okay. We'll get through this."

When they freeze or dissociate: "I'm here. You're in [the kitchen/your room/the car]. You're safe. Can you feel your feet on the floor?"

When they test a boundary repeatedly: "The answer is still the same, and I'm not angry about you asking. It's a no, and I still care about you."

When they have a good moment and then sabotage it: "Good things can feel scary when you're not used to them. That's okay. The good thing is still true, even if it feels weird."

Where We Go From Here

Connection before correction is not a single technique. It is a stance you take toward your child, over and over, in the small moments and the hard ones. It does not eliminate difficult behavior. But it changes the context in which that behavior occurs, from one of power and punishment to one of relationship and repair.

In Chapter 8.0, we go deeper into what your child's behavior is actually saying. You will learn to read the signals underneath the surface and build a practical system for tracking triggers and patterns.

Chapter 8.0 Decoding the Behavior

Your child's behavior is talking to you. Not in words, but in the only language their nervous system knows how to speak. Every meltdown, every shutdown, every instance of hoarding food or refusing touch or lying about something small, these are messages. This chapter teaches you how to read them.

When you can translate your child's behavior into the need or fear underneath it, everything shifts. You stop reacting to the surface and start responding to the source. That shift is the difference between a power struggle and a moment of healing.

The Iceberg Model

Imagine an iceberg. The part above the waterline is what everyone sees: the behavior. The screaming. The lying. The aggression. The refusal. This is what teachers write about in incident reports. It is what family members comment on. It is what makes other parents stare at the grocery store.

Below the waterline is everything that drives the behavior: fear, shame, sensory overload, implicit memories, grief, loneliness, confusion, and the survival responses that were wired into the child's nervous system during years of danger. The visible behavior is never the whole story. It is rarely even the most important part of the story (Beacon House, 2020).

Traditional parenting focuses above the waterline. It sees the behavior and tries to change it directly. Trauma informed parenting looks below the waterline. It asks: what is this behavior trying to accomplish? What does this child need that they cannot ask for with words?

Common Behaviors Decoded

The following section translates the most common CPTSD behaviors into the needs and fears that drive them. Your child may show some of these, all of these, or others not listed here. The principle remains the same: behavior is communication.

Rage and aggression. What it looks like: screaming, hitting, kicking, throwing objects, destroying property. What is underneath: the child's sympathetic nervous system has been activated. They are in fight mode. The rage is not about the spilled juice or the lost toy. It is the body's response to a perceived threat that may be invisible to you (a tone of voice, a facial expression, a sensory trigger). The child feels unsafe and is mobilizing every resource to protect themselves. How to respond: prioritize physical safety, then co-regulate. Do not attempt to reason, lecture, or consequence during the rage. Wait for the thinking brain to come back online (Hughes & Baylin, 2012).

Running and bolting. What it looks like: the child physically flees a situation. They run out of the classroom, out of the house, away from you in a parking lot. What is underneath: flight mode. The nervous system has determined that staying is more dangerous than leaving. The child is not being defiant. They are escaping. The urge to bolt is often triggered by a sudden change, a perceived confrontation, or a sensory overload. How to respond: do not chase aggressively, as this can escalate the flight response. Follow at a safe distance. Use a calm, low voice. When the child stops, give space before approaching.

Dissociation and freezing. What it looks like: the child goes blank. Their eyes glaze over. They do not respond to their name. They may stare at nothing, or appear to be "somewhere else." Some children describe it as watching themselves from outside their body. What is underneath: dorsal vagal shutdown, as we discussed in Chapter 3.0. The nervous system has determined that neither fighting nor fleeing is possible, so it shuts down to conserve resources and reduce pain. This is often mistaken for daydreaming, defiance, or attention deficit. How to respond: grounding techniques. Say the child's name gently. Ask if they can feel their feet on the floor. Offer something with strong sensory input (a cold drink, a textured object). Do not touch without permission. Give time.

Fawning and people pleasing. What it looks like: the child is excessively compliant, agreeable, and focused on keeping adults happy. They apologize constantly, anticipate needs, and suppress their own feelings. What is underneath: the child learned that safety depends on keeping others calm. Any expression of their own needs or preferences risked punishment, so they stopped having visible needs. This is often the most overlooked trauma response because it looks like good behavior. How to respond: gently invite the child's preferences. "What do you actually want?" Normalize disagreement. "It's safe to say no to me." Model that you can handle their displeasure. This takes time, because the child is undoing a survival pattern that may have saved their life (Walker, 2013).

Consider Fenwick (name changed), the eight year old from Chapter 3.0. His adoptive parents initially described him as "the easiest kid." He never argued. He cleaned up without being asked. He thanked them for everything. A trauma informed therapist helped them see the pattern: Fenwick was not easy. He was terrified. His compliance was not comfort. It was a highly refined survival response designed to prevent the adults around him from becoming angry. When his parents began actively encouraging him to express preferences ("It's okay if you don't like the chicken. Tell me what sounds better."), Fenwick initially could not do it. He would freeze, eyes wide, waiting to see if expressing a preference was safe. It took months before he could say, "I don't want peas," without his heart rate visibly increasing.

Hoarding food and objects. What it looks like: the child hides food under their bed, in their closet, or in their backpack. They may collect and guard objects that seem worthless. What is underneath: scarcity programming. The child's early experience taught them that resources are unpredictable. Food disappears. Belongings are taken away. The hoarding is an attempt to create security in the face of perceived scarcity. How to respond: do not punish the behavior. Increase the child's sense of abundance. Keep a snack basket they can access freely. Say, "There will always be enough food in this house. You can have a snack whenever you need one." Allow them to keep a small stash if it provides comfort. Over time, as felt safety builds, the hoarding often decreases naturally (Purvis et al., 2013).

Self harm. What it looks like: hitting themselves, head banging, scratching, picking at skin, or in older children, cutting or burning. What is underneath: the child is trying to manage overwhelming internal pain. Self harm can serve multiple functions. It can bring a dissociated child back to their body. It can release tension from a system locked in hyperarousal. It can provide a sense of control when everything else feels uncontrollable. How to respond: do not react with horror or punishment. Stay calm. Say, "I can see you're hurting. I want to help you find a way to feel better that doesn't hurt your body." Seek professional support immediately. Chapter 12.0 covers crisis response for self harm in detail.

Regression. What it looks like: a child who was functioning at their age level begins behaving like a much younger child. Baby talk, thumb sucking, bedwetting, clinginess, wanting to be carried. What is underneath: stress has overwhelmed the child's capacity to function at their developmental level. Regression is the nervous system's way of returning to a stage where the child felt (or wished they had felt) cared for. How to respond: meet the child where they are. If they need to be held like a younger child, hold them. If they need a bottle or a blanket, provide it. Regression is temporary and is the child's way of asking for nurture they may have missed during the actual developmental window.

Controlling behavior. What it looks like: the child tries to control every aspect of their environment. They dictate seating arrangements, refuse to let others touch their belongings, insist on doing things in a specific order, and become distressed when others deviate from their plan. What is underneath: an attempt to create predictability. The child's early environment was chaotic and uncontrollable. By controlling their current environment, they are trying to prevent the unexpected. How to respond: offer controlled choices within a framework. "You can pick which chair you sit in, and I'm going to decide where the plates go." Provide as much predictability as possible so the child does not need to create it themselves.

Lying. What it looks like: the child lies about things that seem pointless. They deny eating the cookie when there are crumbs on their face. They say they brushed their teeth when they didn't. They fabricate stories about school. What is underneath: lying in traumatized children is almost always a self protection strategy. In their early environment, truth telling may have led to punishment. Or the child may lack the developmental capacity to distinguish between what happened and what they wish had happened. Or they may be testing whether you will become dangerous when you catch them in a lie. How to respond: reduce the stakes. "I think something different happened than what you're telling me, and I'm not angry. Let's figure it out together." Do not corner the child into admitting the lie, as this activates the threat response.

Sexualized behavior. What it looks like: age inappropriate sexual knowledge, language, or behavior. This might include touching others inappropriately, exposing themselves, or mimicking sexual acts. What is underneath: the child may have been exposed to sexual abuse or to adult sexual behavior during their formative years. The behavior does not mean the child is "sexual." It means they were exposed to experiences that should not have happened, and they are processing those experiences in the only way they know how. How to respond: do not shame the child. Calmly redirect: "That's something people do in private" or "That's not something children do." Consult a therapist who specializes in childhood sexual trauma. Chapter 9.0 discusses therapeutic approaches for this and other trauma presentations.

Mapping Your Child's Triggers

A trigger is any stimulus that activates your child's trauma response. Triggers can be sensory (a sound, a smell, a texture), relational (a tone of voice, a facial expression, feeling ignored), situational (transitions, new places, unexpected changes), or temporal (anniversaries of events, certain times of day, specific seasons).

Most parents know some of their child's triggers. But many triggers are hidden, and the only way to identify them is to track the patterns over time.

Consider Larkin (name changed), the 10 year old from Chapter 5.0. His adoptive mother began using a trigger tracking notebook and discovered something unexpected. Larkin's worst days consistently fell on days when his father left for work earlier than usual. The change was only 30 minutes, but it altered the morning routine enough that Larkin's nervous system registered it as unpredictability. Once his parents identified the pattern, they began preparing Larkin the night before ("Dad has an early morning tomorrow, so here's what the morning will look like"). The behavior did not vanish, but it reduced noticeably.

Here is a practical exercise you can use.

For one week, each time your child has a significant behavioral reaction, note the following: the time and place, what happened immediately before the reaction, what the behavior looked like, what you think the child was feeling, and what was happening in the environment (sounds, people present, changes to routine). At the end of the week, look for patterns. You may find that meltdowns cluster around transitions, or that a certain room in the house is consistently the site of difficulty, or that a particular person's presence changes the child's behavior.

Consider Dunstan (name changed), the 15 year old we met in Chapter 2.0. His mother began tracking his behavior and noticed that he was consistently more reactive on Wednesdays. After weeks of tracking, she realized that Wednesday was the day his father had regular phone contact as part of the custody agreement. Even though Dunstan said the calls were "fine," his body was telling a different story. The phone calls were activating his trauma response, and the effects rippled through the rest of the day.

The Behavior Translation Journal

A behavior translation journal is a simple record you keep that helps you practice interpreting your child's behavior through a trauma lens. The format is straightforward.

In one column, write what the child did (the visible behavior). In the next column, write what you think they might have been feeling (the emotion underneath). In the third column, write what the behavior might have been trying to accomplish (the function). And in the fourth column, write what the child might have said if they had the words.

For example. Behavior: threw dinner plate. Feeling: overwhelmed, afraid. Function: ending a situation that felt unsafe. What they would say: "Something about this dinner felt wrong and I needed it to stop."

Behavior: refused to go to school. Feeling: anxious, hypervigilant. Function: avoiding a place that activates the alarm system. What they would say: "School doesn't feel safe and my body won't let me go."

This practice rewires your own responses over time. The more you practice translating behavior into need, the faster you will respond to the need instead of reacting to the behavior. And the more your child feels understood at that level, the less they need the behavior to communicate.

What Comes Next

You now have a working vocabulary for reading your child's behavior. You understand the iceberg model, you can identify common CPTSD behaviors and their underlying drivers, and you have tools for mapping triggers and translating behavior into unspoken needs.

Part Three of this book shifts from daily parenting into the world of treatment: how therapy works for children with CPTSD, how to find the right therapist, and when medication helps. The understanding you have built in Parts One and Two will make you a more informed, effective partner in your child's treatment.

Part Three: The Healing Journey

Therapy, Treatment, and Professional Support

Chapter 9.0 The Therapy Map

Therapy for a child with Complex PTSD is not a single thing. It is a collection of approaches, each designed to address different parts of the damage, delivered in a specific order, by people with specific training. If you have felt overwhelmed by the number of acronyms, modalities, and recommendations thrown at you by providers, school staff, and internet searches, this chapter is designed to cut through that confusion.

By the end, you will understand the major evidence based treatments for childhood CPTSD, how they differ, what each one is best suited for, and what to watch out for when a therapy or practitioner does not meet the standard your child deserves.

Why Order Matters

The most important concept in CPTSD treatment is that it happens in phases. This is not optional. It is the clinical consensus among trauma specialists worldwide, and it has been the standard since Judith Herman first articulated it in 1992 (Herman, 2015).

Phase one is stabilization. Before a child can process what happened to them, they need a foundation of safety, both external (a stable environment, a consistent caregiver) and internal (enough emotional regulation to tolerate distress without falling apart). Phase one focuses on building coping skills, strengthening the relationship between the child and their caregivers, and widening the window of tolerance we discussed in Chapter 3.0. For some children, phase one lasts months. For others, it lasts years. Rushing past it is one of the most common and most damaging mistakes in CPTSD treatment.

Phase two is trauma processing. This is where the child works directly with the traumatic memories, with the support of a trained therapist, to reduce the power those memories hold. The goal is not to erase the past. It is to help the brain file the traumatic experiences into the "past" category so the child's nervous system stops responding as though the danger is still happening.

Phase three is integration and reconnection. The child begins to build a life that is not organized around survival. They develop a more accurate sense of self, form healthier relationships, and expand their capacity for joy, play, and connection (Cloitre et al., 2011).

If a therapist wants to jump straight into trauma processing (asking the child to recount their story, doing exposure exercises, or using EMDR before the child is stabilized), that is a red flag. A child who is pushed into phase two before they are ready can be retraumatized. Their symptoms may worsen. Their trust in therapy may be damaged. And their parents may conclude that therapy does not work, when in fact the therapy was simply delivered out of sequence.

Consider Ivor (name changed), the 11 year old we met in Chapter 4.0. His first therapist, well intentioned but not trained in complex trauma, began asking Ivor to describe his memories of witnessing domestic violence in the second session. Ivor shut down. He refused to return. His parents spent four months rebuilding his willingness to try therapy again. His second therapist spent the first three months playing board games, teaching breathing techniques, and building trust. No trauma was discussed. Ivor's parents were initially frustrated by the slow pace. But the therapist explained: "We're building the container. Without the container, the contents will spill everywhere." When trauma processing eventually began, Ivor was able to tolerate it because the foundation was in place.

Trauma Focused Cognitive Behavioral Therapy

Trauma Focused Cognitive Behavioral Therapy (TF-CBT) is one of the most widely researched treatments for childhood trauma. It was developed by Judith Cohen, Anthony Mannarino, and Esther Deblinger, and it has a strong evidence base for children ages three to 18 who have experienced a range of traumatic events (Cohen et al., 2017).

TF-CBT is structured, typically delivered over 12 to 25 sessions, and it involves both the child and the caregiver. The treatment follows a set of components (often remembered by the acronym PRACTICE): psychoeducation, relaxation skills, affective modulation, cognitive coping, trauma narrative, in vivo mastery, conjoint sessions, and enhancing safety. The caregiver is involved throughout, learning skills in parallel and eventually participating in sessions where the child shares their trauma narrative.

TF-CBT works well for children who have experienced identifiable traumatic events and who have enough stabilization to engage in the structured format. For children with very complex histories, multiple traumas, or severe dissociation, TF-CBT may need to be adapted or combined with other approaches, or preceded by a longer stabilization phase (Cohen et al., 2017).

The ARC Framework

The **Attachment, Regulation, and Competency** (ARC) framework was developed specifically for children with complex trauma. Unlike TF-CBT, which is structured around processing specific traumatic events, ARC is designed to address the broader developmental impact of chronic relational trauma (Blaustein & Kinniburgh, 2018).

ARC focuses on three domains. Attachment addresses the caregiver system, helping parents and providers create safe, attuned relationships. Regulation teaches the child (and the caregiver) skills for managing emotional and physiological arousal. Competency builds the child's sense of self, identity, and agency.

ARC does not follow a rigid session by session protocol. It is a framework that can be adapted to the child's specific needs and pace. This flexibility makes it particularly well suited for children whose trauma histories are complex, layered, and ongoing (such as children still in foster care or children whose family situations are unstable).

Consider Jory (name changed), the 13 year old from Chapter 4.0 who had accumulated five diagnoses without the word "trauma" appearing in any of them. When Jory was finally connected with a therapist trained in the ARC framework, the treatment began with the caregiver system. Jory's mother learned about co-regulation, predictability, and the difference between felt safety and physical safety (concepts from Chapter 6.0). Only after the relational foundation was strengthened did the therapist begin working directly with Jory on regulation and, eventually, on the traumatic memories themselves.

Eye Movement Desensitization and Reprocessing

EMDR (Eye Movement Desensitization and Reprocessing) is a therapeutic approach that uses bilateral stimulation (typically eye movements, but sometimes tapping or auditory tones) to help the brain process traumatic memories. Developed by Francine Shapiro, EMDR has a substantial evidence base for PTSD in both adults and children (Shapiro, 2018).

During EMDR, the child focuses on a traumatic memory while following a bilateral stimulus. The theory is that the bilateral stimulation activates the brain's natural information processing system, allowing the traumatic memory to be integrated into the child's broader memory network. After successful processing, the memory is no longer stored as an active threat. The child can recall it without being flooded by the emotional and physical responses that previously accompanied it.

EMDR can be effective for children with CPTSD, but it requires careful preparation. Because CPTSD involves multiple traumatic memories (not just one), the therapist and child must work together to identify which memories to target and in what order. The stabilization phase is critical. A child who is not adequately stabilized before EMDR may become overwhelmed during processing, which can worsen symptoms rather than improve them.

EMDR has been adapted for use with younger children, incorporating play, drawing, and storytelling to make the process developmentally appropriate. Some children respond very well to EMDR. Others find the bilateral stimulation activating rather than calming. A skilled EMDR therapist will assess the child's readiness and adjust accordingly.

Child Parent Psychotherapy

Child Parent Psychotherapy (CPP) is an evidence based treatment designed specifically for children from birth to age six who have experienced trauma. Developed by Alicia Lieberman, CPP focuses on the relationship between the child and their primary caregiver as the vehicle for healing (Lieberman & Van Horn, 2005).

In CPP, the therapist works with the parent and child together in the room. The therapist helps the parent understand the child's behavior through a trauma lens, supports the parent in responding to the child's cues, and facilitates moments of connection and repair. For very young children, who cannot articulate their experiences in words, CPP uses play, narrative, and the caregiver's attuned presence to process traumatic experiences.

CPP is particularly valuable for families formed through adoption or foster care, where the caregiver relationship is new and the child's attachment patterns were shaped by previous harmful relationships. It is also used with biological families where trauma has disrupted the parent child bond.

Consider Hadrian (name changed), the six year old from Chapter 3.0 who screamed when his foster father cooked with onions. His therapist used CPP to help the foster family understand Hadrian's implicit memories and to build attuned responses. Over time, the foster father learned to narrate cooking activities in advance ("I'm going to use onions tonight. They might smell strong."), which gave Hadrian's nervous system a chance to prepare rather than be ambushed by the sensory trigger.

Play Therapy and Expressive Arts

Not all children can engage in talk based therapy, especially young children, nonverbal children, and children whose trauma occurred before they had language. For these children, **play therapy** and **expressive arts therapies** offer an alternative pathway to processing.

In play therapy, the therapist creates a safe environment with carefully selected toys and materials. The child plays, and the therapist observes, reflects, and gently guides the play toward themes related to the child's experience. Through play, children can enact, process, and master experiences that they cannot put into words. A child who repeatedly crashes toy cars may be processing a frightening event. A child who buries dolls in sand may be expressing something about loss or concealment (Landreth, 2012).

Expressive arts therapies (art, music, movement, drama) work on a similar principle. They give the child a medium for expression that bypasses the verbal centers of the brain and accesses the body based, sensory, and emotional channels where trauma is stored (as we discussed in Chapter 3.0).

These approaches are often used during the stabilization phase or as a complement to other treatments. They are particularly effective for children whose trauma occurred in the preverbal period, for children who dissociate during talk therapy, and for children who resist structured approaches.

Somatic Approaches

Because CPTSD lives in the body as much as the mind (Chapter 3.0), treatments that address the body's stress response directly are increasingly recognized as valuable. **Somatic experiencing**, developed by Peter Levine, helps the child discharge the physical energy trapped in the nervous system by traumatic events. **Sensory motor psychotherapy** works with body posture, movement, and sensation to process trauma stored below conscious awareness (Levine & Kline, 2007).

These approaches are particularly useful for children who hold their trauma in physical symptoms: chronic pain, tension, startle responses, and sensory sensitivities. They are typically used alongside (not instead of) other treatments.

DBT for Adolescents

Dialectical Behavior Therapy (DBT) was originally developed for adults with borderline personality disorder, but adapted versions have been shown to be effective for adolescents with emotional dysregulation, self harm, and suicidal ideation (Miller et al., 2007).

DBT teaches four core skill sets: mindfulness, distress tolerance, emotion regulation, and interpersonal effectiveness. For teenagers with CPTSD, who often struggle with all four of these areas, DBT provides concrete, practicable skills that can be used in daily life. It also includes a family component, which teaches parents and teens shared language and strategies.

DBT is not a standalone treatment for CPTSD. It does not include trauma processing. But it is an excellent stabilization tool, especially for teens who are self harming, struggling with substance use, or experiencing intense emotional volatility.

Consider Dunstan (name changed), the 15 year old from Chapter 2.0 who had been caught stealing. His therapist recommended a

DBT skills group as the first phase of treatment. The group taught Dunstan distress tolerance skills he could use when his nervous system was overwhelmed, and it gave him language for emotional states he had never been able to name. After six months of DBT, his therapist introduced trauma processing work. The DBT skills became the foundation that made the processing possible.

Emerging Approaches

Neurofeedback uses real time monitoring of brain activity to help children learn to regulate their own neural patterns. The child watches a screen while sensors on their scalp measure brainwave activity. When the brain produces the desired pattern (such as calm, focused states), the screen responds positively. Over time, the brain learns to produce these patterns more consistently. Research on neurofeedback for PTSD is growing, with some promising results, though the evidence base is not yet as strong as for TF-CBT or EMDR (van der Kolk et al., 2016).

Other emerging approaches include **yoga and mindfulness based interventions** (which help regulate the body's stress response), **equine assisted therapy** (which uses the relationship with horses to build trust, attunement, and regulation), and **internal family systems** (IFS) therapy, which helps children understand and work with different "parts" of themselves. Each of these has clinical support but varying levels of rigorous research evidence.

When evaluating any treatment, ask: Is there published research supporting this approach for children with complex trauma? Is the practitioner trained and supervised? Is the treatment being delivered in the right phase (stabilization vs. processing)? And is my child responding positively over time?

What to Watch Out For

Not all therapies are created equal, and not all practitioners are adequately trained. Here are warning signs that a therapy or therapist may not be appropriate for your child.

A therapist who pushes into trauma processing before the child is stabilized. A practitioner who uses confrontational techniques, raised voices, or physical restraint as part of "therapy." Any approach that promises rapid results (such as "your child will be healed in three sessions"). Therapies that rely on breaking the child's will, enforcing compliance through withholding affection, or using the child's attachment needs against them. Any practice that discourages the caregiver's involvement or refuses to communicate with you about your child's treatment (with appropriate confidentiality for older children).

Holding therapy, rebirthing therapy, and any modality that involves physical coercion have been associated with harm and even death in children. These practices are condemned by every major professional organization in the field of child psychology and should be avoided absolutely (Chaffin et al., 2006).

Making Sense of It All

The number of therapeutic approaches can feel overwhelming. Here is a simplified way to think about it. Stabilization first, always. TF-CBT, ARC, and CPP are well established for children with CPTSD. EMDR is a strong option for processing once the child is stable. Play therapy and somatic work are valuable throughout, especially for younger children. DBT is excellent for teens who need regulation skills before processing. Emerging approaches can complement but should not replace established treatments.

In Chapter 10.0, we move from understanding the options to finding the right person to deliver them. You will learn what credentials to look for, what questions to ask, and how to build a treatment team that works for your child.

Chapter 10.0 Finding the Right Therapist

Knowing what kind of therapy your child needs is one thing. Finding the person who can deliver it is another. This chapter is a practical guide to identifying, evaluating, and working with the right therapist for your child. It also addresses the realities that make the search difficult: waitlists, insurance limitations, geographic barriers, and the exhaustion of advocating for your child while you are already running on empty.

What Training Actually Matters

Not all therapists are trained to work with Complex PTSD in children. A therapist may be licensed, experienced, and well intentioned, but if they have not received specific training in developmental trauma, they may not recognize CPTSD, may apply inappropriate interventions, or may inadvertently retraumatize your child.

Here is what to look for. First, the therapist should have a license in a mental health discipline: Licensed Clinical Social Worker (LCSW), Licensed Professional Counselor (LPC), Licensed Marriage and Family Therapist (LMFT), or a psychologist (PhD or PsyD). Licensure is the baseline. It tells you the person has met their state's requirements for education and supervised practice. But licensure alone does not guarantee trauma competence.

Second, look for specific training in one or more of the evidence based approaches described in Chapter 9.0. TF-CBT certification requires completion of a structured training program with ongoing consultation. EMDR certification (through EMDRIA) requires both training and supervised clinical hours. Clinicians trained in the ARC framework, CPP, or DBT will typically list these in their professional profiles or on their practice websites.

Ask directly. A therapist who is vague about their trauma training may not have received any.

Third, look for experience with the population your child belongs to. A therapist who specializes in single incident trauma (car accidents, natural disasters) may not be equipped for the layered, relational trauma that defines CPTSD. A therapist who primarily works with adults may not be equipped for the developmental considerations of treating children. And a therapist who works mainly with adolescents may not be the right fit for a five year old. Specificity matters.

Consider Elowen (name changed), the foster mother from Chapter 1.0. She described calling six therapists before finding one who could work with her daughter. "The first two had never heard of CPTSD. The third said she treated 'anxiety and depression in children' but not trauma specifically. The fourth had a six month waitlist. The fifth only took one insurance plan we didn't have. The sixth was the right person, and I almost didn't have the energy to make the call."

Elowen's experience is common. The search itself is draining, and it often happens at a time when parents are already depleted. But the right therapist makes a difference that justifies the effort.

Questions for the First Phone Call

Before scheduling an intake appointment, most therapists will offer a brief phone consultation (typically 10 to 15 minutes). This is your chance to assess fit. Here are the questions to ask.

What is your training and experience with complex trauma in children? (You are looking for specifics: named modalities, certification status, years of experience with this population.)

Are you familiar with the ICD-11 definition of CPTSD and the concept of Developmental Trauma Disorder? (This tells you whether the therapist's framework extends beyond the DSM-5.)

How do you approach the early sessions with a traumatized child? (You are listening for language about stabilization, relationship building, and phase based treatment. A therapist who describes jumping quickly into "talking about what happened" may not be operating within the recommended sequence.)

How do you involve caregivers in treatment? (For children with CPTSD, caregiver involvement is essential. A therapist who works exclusively behind closed doors, without any communication with you, is missing a critical component.)

What does progress look like in your experience, and what is a realistic timeline? (This helps you calibrate expectations. A therapist who promises rapid results or who cannot articulate what progress looks like may not have sufficient experience.)

How do you handle crises between sessions? (Children with CPTSD may have crises that cannot wait for the next appointment. You need to know whether the therapist has a plan for this.)

Do you coordinate with schools, psychiatrists, or other providers? (Complex trauma often requires a team approach. A therapist who works in isolation may not be meeting all of your child's needs.)

Your Role in Therapy

Your involvement in your child's therapy will depend on the child's age, the therapeutic modality, and the therapist's approach. In general, parents of younger children (under 12) are more actively involved. Therapies like CPP and TF-CBT have built in caregiver components. You may participate directly in sessions, learn skills in parallel, or join for specific activities.

For older children and adolescents, the therapist may work primarily with the teen and meet with you separately or periodically. Confidentiality becomes more important as children age, and your teen may need a space where they can speak freely without worrying about your reaction.

Regardless of the format, you should expect regular communication with the therapist about your child's progress, the treatment plan, and any adjustments. You should feel that your observations are valued, because you see your child in contexts the therapist never will. And you should feel comfortable asking questions without being dismissed.

Consider Crispin (name changed), the 12 year old from Chapter 2.0. His foster parents initially felt shut out of therapy. The therapist met with Crispin weekly but rarely communicated with them. After three months, the foster parents requested a meeting and asked how they could support the work at home. The therapist, to his credit, adjusted his approach and began scheduling monthly parent sessions. "Once we were part of the process," the foster father said, "everything moved faster. We could reinforce what he was learning. We could see the patterns."

If you feel excluded from your child's treatment and your requests for involvement are repeatedly dismissed, it may be time to discuss this concern directly with the therapist, or to consider whether a different therapist would be a better fit.

When to Stay and When to Switch

Therapy is not always comfortable, and discomfort does not automatically mean the therapy is wrong. Your child may resist going. They may have harder days after sessions, especially as they begin processing difficult material. They may say they hate therapy. These reactions can be normal parts of the process.

However, there are signs that the therapy is not working or is causing harm. If your child's symptoms are consistently worsening over a period of months (not just temporary spikes after hard sessions, but a sustained downward trend). If your child is being retraumatized in sessions (coming home in states of dissociation, panic, or shutdown that were not present before therapy began). If the therapist dismisses your concerns or refuses to explain their approach. If the therapist uses techniques that are coercive, confrontational, or physically restraining. Any of these warrant a conversation, and potentially a change.

Switching therapists is not failure. It is advocacy. The therapeutic relationship matters enormously, and a child who does not feel safe with their therapist will not benefit from the treatment, no matter how evidence based the modality.

Consider Kenrick (name changed), the nine year old from Chapter 4.0 who had both ADHD and CPTSD. His first therapist focused exclusively on behavioral strategies for the ADHD, ignoring the trauma history entirely. After six months of minimal progress, Kenrick's parents sought a second opinion from a trauma specialist, who restructured the treatment plan to address both conditions. "I felt guilty leaving the first therapist," Kenrick's mother said. "But my son needed someone who could see the whole picture."

Insurance, Waitlists, and Access

The practical barriers to accessing quality trauma therapy are real and significant. Here is how to work with them.

Insurance. Many trauma specialists do not accept insurance, which creates an immediate financial barrier. If your insurance plan has out of network benefits, you may be able to seek reimbursement for a portion of the cost. Ask the therapist for a superbill (a receipt with diagnostic and procedure codes) that you can submit to your insurance. If your child is on Medicaid, look for community mental health centers that employ trauma trained clinicians. Some states have Medicaid waivers that cover intensive therapeutic services for children with trauma histories.

Waitlists. Demand for qualified trauma therapists exceeds supply in most areas. If the therapist you want has a waitlist, get on it, but do not wait passively. Ask if they can recommend a colleague with similar training. Ask if they offer group therapy or parent consultation while you wait. And look into the other modalities described in Chapter 9.0 that might bridge the gap (play therapy, DBT skills groups, somatic work).

Telehealth. The expansion of telehealth services has improved access for families in rural or underserved areas. Many evidence based treatments for childhood CPTSD can be delivered effectively via video, though some components (particularly play therapy for young children and EMDR for certain clients) may require in person sessions. If your area lacks trauma specialists, a telehealth provider in another part of your state may be an option.

Geographic barriers. If you live in an area with few mental health providers, consider whether a periodic intensive model might work. Some clinics offer concentrated treatment blocks (such as weekly sessions over a two week period) followed by less frequent maintenance sessions. This can reduce the burden of long distance travel.

Building a Treatment Team

Your child's needs may extend beyond what any single therapist can provide. A treatment team might include a therapist for individual trauma work, a family therapist to support the caregiver child relationship, a psychiatrist for medication management (discussed in Chapter 11.0), an occupational therapist for sensory processing support, and a school based counselor who coordinates with the clinical team.

You are the hub of this team. You are the person who carries information between providers, who notices when one part of the treatment plan conflicts with another, and who advocates for your child when the professionals do not communicate with each other.

This is exhausting work. It should not fall entirely on you, and in an ideal system, it would not. But in the system as it exists, informed and persistent parent advocacy is often what holds the treatment together. Chapter 17.0 addresses how to build support around yourself so that you are not carrying this alone.

Consider Oswin (name changed), the 14 year old from Chapter 5.0 whose behavior at school and home were dramatically different. His treatment team eventually included a trauma therapist, a DBT skills group, a psychiatrist, and a school counselor who met monthly with his foster parents. "It took us almost a year to assemble the team," his foster mother said. "But once everyone was talking to each other, the progress was visible. No one person could have done what the team did together."

Getting Started

If your child is not currently in therapy and you are unsure where to begin, start with one step. Call your pediatrician and ask for a referral to a trauma trained therapist. Search the provider directories of the National Child Traumatic Stress Network (NCTSN), Psychology Today (filtering for "trauma" and your child's age), or the EMDR International Association. Ask other parents in support groups for adoptive, foster, or kinship families for recommendations.

The goal is not to find the perfect therapist on the first try. The goal is to begin. In Chapter 11.0, we turn to the question parents often ask alongside therapy: does my child need medication, and how do I make that decision wisely?

Chapter 11.0 Medication Conversations

Medication is one of the most charged topics in parenting a child with CPTSD. Some parents arrive at the question already having been told by a provider that their child needs medication. Others arrive because nothing else has worked and they are desperate for something to help. Still others resist the idea entirely, worried about side effects, dependency, or the message it sends.

This chapter is not here to tell you whether your child should take medication. That decision belongs to you, your child's prescriber, and (when age appropriate) your child. What this chapter will do is give you the information you need to participate in that decision as an informed partner, to ask the right questions, and to monitor the results.

When Medication Helps

Medication does not treat CPTSD. There is no pill that addresses the three core pillars described in Chapter 2.0: emotional dysregulation, negative self concept, and disturbed relationships. Those require relational, therapeutic, and developmental interventions over time. What medication can do is reduce specific symptoms enough that the child can engage in therapy, stay in school, sleep through the night, or get through the day without being overwhelmed by their own nervous system .

Think of medication as scaffolding, not as the building. The building is therapy, relationship, and developmental growth. The scaffolding supports the construction by managing the symptoms that would otherwise make the work impossible.

There are situations where medication is worth considering. When a child's anxiety is so severe that they cannot participate in therapy. When sleep disruption is so persistent that the child is chronically exhausted and unable to function during the day. When hyperarousal is so intense that the child is in a near constant state of fight or flight, unable to access their thinking brain even in safe environments. When depression has settled so deeply that the child has lost interest in everything and is struggling to engage with the world at all. And when self harm or suicidal thoughts are present and creating immediate safety concerns.

In each of these cases, medication is not solving the problem. It is turning down the volume enough that other interventions can reach the child.

Consider Godric (name changed), the 10 year old from Chapter 3.0 who cycled between three nervous system states. His therapist had been working with him for six months, but progress was stalled. Godric's hyperarousal was so intense that he could not stay in his window of tolerance long enough to practice the skills his therapist was teaching. A child psychiatrist started a low dose of an alpha-2 agonist (a medication that reduces the body's stress response). Within three weeks, Godric's mother noticed that the peaks were less extreme. He was still having hard moments, but he was coming back from them faster. "The medication didn't fix him," she said. "It gave him enough room to let the therapy in."

The Problem with Medicating the Diagnosis

One of the most common pitfalls in medicating children with CPTSD is that prescribers treat the diagnostic label rather than the symptom pattern. As we discussed in Chapter 4.0, children with CPTSD are frequently diagnosed with ADHD, bipolar disorder, ODD, or anxiety disorders. When those labels are treated pharmacologically without considering the underlying trauma, the results can be disappointing or harmful.

A child who is diagnosed with ADHD based on trauma driven hypervigilance may be prescribed stimulant medication.

Stimulants increase arousal. For a child whose nervous system is already in overdrive, this can intensify anxiety, agitation, and meltdowns rather than improving focus. The medication is treating the wrong mechanism.

A child who is diagnosed with bipolar disorder based on trauma driven emotional swings may be prescribed mood stabilizers or atypical antipsychotics. These medications carry significant side effects (weight gain, metabolic changes, sedation) and may not address the actual problem, which is a dysregulated stress response, not a mood cycling disorder.

A child who is diagnosed with ODD may be prescribed nothing at all, because ODD is typically treated with behavioral interventions. Meanwhile, the child's underlying anxiety, hyperarousal, and trauma responses go unaddressed.

The key question to ask any prescriber is: Are we treating the diagnosis, or are we treating the symptoms? A thoughtful prescriber will be able to explain which specific symptoms they are targeting with a medication and how they will measure whether the medication is working.

Consider Jory (name changed), the 13 year old from Chapter 4.0 with five accumulated diagnoses. Over the course of four years, Jory had been prescribed a stimulant for ADHD, a mood stabilizer for "rule out bipolar," and an SSRI for anxiety. He was on three medications simultaneously, none of which were prescribed with his trauma history in mind. When his trauma focused therapist coordinated with a new psychiatrist who understood CPTSD, the medications were gradually adjusted. The stimulant was removed (his attention problems were driven by hyperarousal, not ADHD). The mood stabilizer was tapered. A low dose of an SSRI was maintained because it was helping with his anxiety baseline. The reduction from three medications to one, combined with trauma therapy, produced more improvement in six months than the previous four years of polypharmacy had.

Questions to Ask Before Starting Medication

Before agreeing to any psychotropic medication for your child, bring these questions to the prescribing physician or psychiatrist.

What specific symptoms are we targeting with this medication? (The answer should be concrete: sleep, hyperarousal, anxiety, concentration. If the answer is "the ADHD" or "the bipolar," press further. You need symptom level specificity.)

Has my child's trauma history been considered in this recommendation? (If the prescriber is not aware of your child's trauma history, provide it. If they are aware but do not factor it into their prescribing rationale, that is a concern.)

What are the expected benefits and the timeline for seeing them? (Most psychiatric medications take two to six weeks to show full effects. A prescriber who promises immediate results or cannot articulate when you should expect to see change may not be giving you realistic information.)

What are the potential side effects, and how will we monitor for them? (Every medication has a side effect profile. You should know what to watch for and have a plan for regular check ins.)

How does this medication interact with my child's current medications, if any? (Drug interactions can be significant, especially in children on multiple prescriptions.)

What is the plan if this medication does not work? (A thoughtful prescriber will have a contingency plan and will not simply add another medication on top of a failing one.)

Is this medication being used off label, and if so, what is the evidence for this use in children? (Many psychiatric medications used in children are prescribed off label, meaning they are approved for adults but not specifically for children. This is not inherently wrong, but you deserve to know.)

What is the plan for eventual discontinuation? (Most psychiatric medications for children are not intended to be permanent. Ask about the long term plan from the beginning.)

Common Medication Categories

The following overview describes the medication classes most commonly used for symptoms associated with CPTSD in children. This is not prescriptive guidance. It is information to help you understand what a prescriber may recommend and why.

SSRIs (selective serotonin reuptake inhibitors, such as sertraline and fluoxetine) are commonly prescribed for anxiety and depression in children. They can help reduce the emotional intensity and fearfulness that accompany CPTSD. Side effects may include nausea, headache, changes in appetite, and in some cases, increased agitation in the initial weeks. The FDA has issued a black box warning regarding a potential increased risk of suicidal ideation in children and adolescents on SSRIs, which requires careful monitoring .

Alpha-2 agonists (such as guanfacine and clonidine) are used to reduce hyperarousal and improve sleep. These medications work by dampening the body's stress response, which can help a chronically activated child come closer to baseline. Side effects may include drowsiness, dizziness, and low blood pressure. These medications are sometimes a better first choice than stimulants for children whose attention difficulties are driven by trauma rather than ADHD.

Atypical antipsychotics (such as risperidone and aripiprazole) are sometimes prescribed for severe aggression or emotional volatility. They carry significant metabolic side effects and should generally be reserved for cases where other approaches have not been sufficient. Regular monitoring of weight, blood sugar, and lipid levels is recommended.

Stimulants (such as methylphenidate and amphetamine based medications) are the standard treatment for ADHD but should be used cautiously in children with CPTSD. In some cases, a child may have genuine co-occurring ADHD that benefits from stimulant treatment. In other cases, stimulants may worsen trauma related hyperarousal. Careful diagnostic clarity (Chapter 4.0) is essential before starting a stimulant.

Melatonin is an over the counter supplement commonly used to help children with CPTSD fall asleep. Sleep disruption is one of the most pervasive symptoms of complex trauma, and melatonin can support the body's natural sleep cycle with a relatively favorable side effect profile. It is not a sedative and works best when combined with consistent bedtime routines and a sensory appropriate sleep environment (as described in Chapter 6.0).

Monitoring What Happens

Once your child starts a medication, your observations become critical data. Keep a simple log of what you notice: changes in sleep, appetite, mood, energy, behavior, and physical symptoms. Note improvements as well as concerns. Bring this log to every medication management appointment.

Consider Larkin (name changed), the 10 year old from Chapter 5.0. When his prescriber started him on an SSRI for anxiety, his adoptive mother began keeping a daily log. She noticed that while his anxiety decreased noticeably in the first three weeks, he also became more emotionally flat, losing interest in activities he had previously enjoyed. She brought this to the prescriber, who adjusted the dosage. The flatness resolved, and the anxiety reduction was maintained at the lower dose. Without her observations, the side effect might have been missed.

Medication and Therapy Together

The research is consistent: for children with CPTSD, the best outcomes come from combining appropriate medication with trauma focused therapy, not from either one alone. Medication manages symptoms. Therapy addresses root causes. The two approaches complement each other when they are coordinated.

This requires that your child's prescriber and therapist communicate with each other. Ask both providers whether they are willing to be in contact. Share information between them yourself if necessary. The prescriber needs to know what is happening in therapy (for example, if the child is entering a more activating phase of trauma processing, the prescriber may want to monitor more closely). The therapist needs to know what medications the child is on and how they are responding.

Consider Fenwick (name changed), the eight year old from Chapter 3.0. His treatment plan included both a trauma therapist and a child psychiatrist. When his therapist began incorporating more active trauma processing, she alerted the psychiatrist, who slightly increased Fenwick's nighttime dose of guanfacine to support his sleep during the more activating therapy phase. This kind of coordination is what integrated care looks like.

Trusting Your Instincts

You know your child better than any provider. If a medication does not feel right, if your child's personality seems to vanish, if the side effects seem worse than the symptoms, if you are being pressured to add more medications without clear justification, trust what you are seeing. You have the right to ask questions, to seek second opinions, and to say no.

At the same time, try not to let fear prevent your child from receiving help they genuinely need. Some children benefit enormously from the right medication at the right dose. The goal is not to avoid medication at all costs. The goal is to use it thoughtfully, as one tool within a broader plan, with your child's full picture in view.

Moving Forward

Parts One through Three of this book have given you a foundation: understanding what CPTSD is, how it affects your child's brain, how to parent differently, and how to navigate therapy and medication. In Part Four, we turn to the hardest moments: crises, school battles, family impact, and the systems your family must navigate. The understanding you have built will carry you through.

Part Four: The Hard Parts

Navigating Crisis, School, Siblings, and Systems

Chapter 12.0 When Crisis Hits

There will be moments when everything you have learned in this book narrows to a single point: your child is in crisis, and you need to know what to do right now. This chapter is written for those moments. It covers trauma triggered meltdowns, dissociative episodes, self harm, and situations where safety is at immediate risk. It also covers what happens after the crisis passes, because the repair matters as much as the response.

If you are reading this chapter in the middle of a crisis, skip to the section that matches what is happening. You can come back and read the rest later.

Meltdown vs. Tantrum

The distinction matters because the response is different. A tantrum is goal directed. The child wants something, and the tantrum is the strategy to get it. A tantrum typically escalates when the child has an audience and de-escalates when the audience leaves or when the goal is either met or clearly unattainable. The child maintains some awareness of their surroundings and some capacity for decision making during a tantrum.

A **trauma triggered meltdown** is not goal directed. It is the nervous system's involuntary response to a perceived threat. The child is not trying to get something. They are reacting to something their body interprets as dangerous, even if the actual situation is safe. During a meltdown, the thinking brain is offline. The child cannot hear reason, process consequences, or make strategic decisions. They are in survival mode (Perry & Szalavitz, 2006).

You can usually tell the difference by asking yourself: Does this behavior have an audience? If I leave the room, does it escalate or wind down? Is the child aware of what they are doing, or do they seem lost in it? Is there a demand attached, or is this pure distress?

If it is a tantrum, standard parenting strategies (acknowledging the feeling, holding the limit, waiting it out) can work. If it is a trauma triggered meltdown, those strategies will likely fail, because the child is not operating from the part of their brain that responds to logic or social pressure.

De-Escalation by Response Type

The nervous system states described in Chapter 3.0 (fight, flight, freeze, fawn, and collapse) each require a different response. Using the wrong approach for the wrong state can make things worse.

When the child is in fight mode (screaming, hitting, kicking, throwing, destroying): Your first priority is physical safety. Move other people and breakable objects out of range. Do not try to physically restrain the child unless they are about to seriously injure themselves or someone else, because physical restraint often escalates the fight response. Lower your body position. Speak in short, calm phrases: "I'm here. You're safe. I'm going to stay right here." Do not lecture, reason, or ask questions. The thinking brain cannot process any of it. Wait for the wave to crest. It will. When the intensity begins to drop, offer something grounding: a drink of water, a blanket, a move to a quieter space. Do not attempt to discuss the episode until the child is fully regulated, which may be hours later (Hughes & Baylin, 2012).

When the child is in flight mode (running, bolting, trying to escape): Do not chase aggressively. Pursuit activates the flight response further. Follow at a safe distance. If the child is heading toward danger (a street, an open window), intervene physically with the minimum force necessary to prevent harm. If they are running within a safe space, let them move. Movement discharges the energy of sympathetic activation. When they slow or stop, approach slowly and from an angle rather than head on.

Say their name gently. Offer a choice: "Do you want to sit here or go inside?"

When the child is in freeze or collapse (glazed eyes, unresponsive, staring, limp body): This is dorsal vagal shutdown. The child has left the present moment. Do not shout, shake, or try to snap them out of it. Speak slowly and gently. Use their name. Offer sensory anchors: "Can you feel your feet on the floor? Can you hear my voice? You are in the kitchen. It is Tuesday." Offer something with strong sensory input if they are able to receive it (a cold glass of water, a textured object to hold, a weighted blanket). Give time. Coming out of a freeze state can take minutes, and rushing the process can push the child back into it.

Consider Godric (name changed), the 10 year old from Chapter 3.0 whose mother described his "three settings." During one episode, Godric went from screaming (fight) to running to his room (flight) to sitting motionless on his bed staring at the wall (freeze) in the space of 12 minutes. His mother, who had learned about nervous system states from his therapist, matched her response to each shift. She stayed calm and present during the screaming. She let him run but followed. When he froze, she sat on the floor outside his room and said, "I'm right here, Godric. You're in your bedroom. You're safe. I'm going to stay." After eight minutes, he blinked, looked at her, and said, "Can I have some water?" The crisis was over. The repair could begin.

Grounding for Dissociation

Dissociation is one of the most frightening experiences for a parent to witness. Your child is physically present but mentally absent. They may not respond to their name. Their eyes may be open but unfocused. They may appear to be looking through you rather than at you. Some children describe it afterward as "going somewhere else" or "watching from far away."

Dissociation is not the child being dramatic or ignoring you. It is the nervous system's protective shutdown, as described in

Chapter 3.0. The brain has determined that the current experience is too overwhelming to process, and it reduces awareness to protect the child from pain.

Grounding techniques work by gently bringing the child's awareness back to the present through sensory input. Here are several you can use.

Name and orient. Say the child's name. Tell them where they are. "Hadrian, you're in the living room. It is Saturday afternoon. You are safe. I am here with you." Repeat calmly.

Engage the senses. Ask the child to name five things they can see, four they can touch, three they can hear, two they can smell, and one they can taste. If they cannot speak, offer the sensory input directly: place a cold cloth on their wrist, offer a piece of ice to hold, play a familiar song quietly.

Ground through the body. Ask the child to press their feet into the floor. To squeeze their hands together. To wiggle their toes. Physical sensation helps reconnect the mind to the body.

Do not touch without warning. For a dissociating child, unexpected physical contact can feel threatening and deepen the dissociation. Always announce before touching: "I'm going to put my hand on your shoulder, okay?"

Consider Hadrian (name changed), the six year old from Chapter 3.0. When he dissociated, his foster father learned to sit nearby, speak his name softly, and offer a cup of warm water (which provided temperature sensation and something to hold). "The first time it happened, I panicked," his foster father said. "I thought something was medically wrong. Once I understood it was dissociation, I could respond instead of react. The warm water became our thing. He would hold it with both hands and slowly come back."

Responding to Self Harm

If your child is engaging in self harm (hitting themselves, scratching, picking skin, cutting, burning, head banging), the first and most important thing is to stay calm. Your visible distress, however natural it is, can increase the child's shame and escalate the behavior.

Self harm in traumatized children serves multiple functions, as discussed in Chapter 8.0. It may release overwhelming internal pressure. It may bring a dissociated child back into their body. It may provide a sense of control when everything else feels uncontrollable. Understanding the function is important, but in the moment of crisis, the priority is safety, not analysis.

Remove access to means of harm if you can do so safely (take away sharp objects, move the child away from walls they are hitting). Do not grab or restrain unless absolutely necessary. Say: "I can see you're hurting. I want to help. Can we find a way that doesn't hurt your body?" Offer an alternative: squeezing ice cubes (the intensity of sensation without lasting harm), tearing paper or cardboard, pressing hands against a wall with maximum effort, stomping feet hard on the floor.

After the immediate danger has passed, this is not the time for a conversation about why self harm is wrong. The child already knows. What they need is to hear: "I'm not angry. I'm not scared of you. I want to help you find safer ways to manage this pain."

Self harm always warrants professional involvement. If your child is actively self harming and does not have a therapist, this is the time to seek one. If they do have a therapist, contact the therapist promptly to update the treatment plan. If the self harm is severe or escalating, or if the child expresses intent to die, go to the nearest emergency department or call 988 (Suicide and Crisis Lifeline in the United States).

Safety Planning

A safety plan is a document you create in advance, during a calm time, that tells everyone in the household what to do when a crisis happens. You do not want to be making decisions about who to call and what to do while your child is in the middle of a meltdown. You want those decisions already made.

A safety plan includes the following. Names and phone numbers of your child's therapist, psychiatrist, and pediatrician. The local crisis line number and the national 988 number. The address of the nearest emergency department. A list of de-escalation strategies that work for your child (you will build this over time through trial and observation). A plan for keeping other family members safe during a crisis (who takes the siblings to another room, who stays with the child in crisis). A plan for what to do if the child needs to be transported to an emergency facility. Any medications the child takes, listed with dosages, in case emergency providers need the information.

Post this plan somewhere accessible (the refrigerator, a folder in the kitchen, a note in your phone). Make sure every adult in the household knows where it is and what it says. Review it periodically and update it as your child's needs change.

Consider Elowen (name changed), the foster mother from Chapter 1.0. After a particularly severe meltdown during which her daughter tried to leave the house at night, Elowen worked with her daughter's therapist to create a family crisis plan. "Having it written down changed everything," she said. "Not because the crises stopped, but because I stopped freezing during them. I had a plan. I could follow the steps instead of panicking."

Post Crisis Repair

After a crisis, both you and your child need repair. The crisis itself is the wave. The repair is what determines whether the wave leaves damage or deposits something useful.

Wait until the child is fully regulated before attempting repair. This might be 30 minutes after a meltdown or several hours after a severe episode. You will know they are ready when their voice, face, and body return to baseline.

Repair sounds like: "That was really hard. I'm glad we got through it." Not: "Let's talk about what you did." You can gently name what you observed: "It looked like something really scared you." You can ask an open question: "Is there anything you want me to know about what happened?" But do not push. Some children will want to process verbally. Others will not, and that is fine. The repair is in the reconnection, not the conversation.

If you lost your temper during the crisis (you raised your voice, you said something sharp, you grabbed the child when you didn't need to), own it. "I got scared, and I yelled. That wasn't okay. I'm sorry. I'm going to work on that." This models the rupture and repair cycle described in Chapter 7.0, and it teaches the child that adults can make mistakes without becoming permanently dangerous.

Consider Bramwell (name changed), the kinship caregiver from Chapter 1.0. After a meltdown during which he raised his voice at his niece, he felt terrible. His instinct was to pretend it didn't happen. But his niece's therapist coached him to address it directly. The next morning, he sat with his niece and said, "I yelled last night, and I'm sorry. You were having a hard time, and my job was to stay calm, and I didn't. That wasn't your fault." His niece looked at him for a long time. Then she said, "It's okay. You came back." Four words that told him the repair had landed.

Where This Leads

Crises are inevitable when you are raising a child with CPTSD. What is not inevitable is how you respond to them. With preparation, understanding, and the willingness to repair, each crisis can become an opportunity to teach your child's nervous system something new: that the adults in their life can handle the hard moments without becoming dangerous, disappearing, or falling apart.

In Chapter 13.0, we move from the home to the school, where a different kind of crisis often unfolds: the daily struggle to get your child's educational needs met in a system that was not built for them.

Chapter 13.0 Advocating at School

School is where the gap between what your child needs and what the system provides becomes most visible. Your child spends six to eight hours a day in an environment designed for children whose nervous systems function within a predictable range. The expectations of school (sit still, follow directions, transition smoothly, manage frustration quietly, interact with peers, tolerate noise and crowding) read like a list of the things CPTSD makes hardest.

This chapter gives you the knowledge and tools to advocate effectively for your child's educational needs. It covers trauma informed education, the legal frameworks that can protect your child, specific accommodations that make a difference, and what to do when the school system responds to your child's trauma with punishment instead of support.

Why School Is So Hard

Before we talk about advocacy, it helps to understand why school is often the setting where your child's symptoms are most visible. Everything about the typical school environment can activate a traumatized child's nervous system.

The noise level in a cafeteria or gymnasium can overwhelm a child whose sensory system is already hypervigilant. Transitions between activities require the kind of cognitive flexibility that depends on prefrontal cortex function, which may be compromised (Chapter 3.0). Being told what to do by authority figures can trigger survival responses in a child who learned that compliance with adults led to harm. Peer conflict, even minor, can feel like a threat. And the structure of the school day (with its rigid schedule, performance expectations, and social demands) leaves almost no room for the kind of decompression a traumatized child needs.

Consider Ivor (name changed), the 11 year old from Chapter 4.0. His school reported that he was "constantly disruptive," leaving his seat, arguing with teachers, and getting into conflicts with peers. The school's response was escalating consequences: verbal warnings, loss of recess, in school suspension. Each consequence increased Ivor's distress, which increased the disruptive behavior, which led to more consequences. By the time his parents requested a meeting, Ivor had received 14 disciplinary referrals in a single semester.

Ivor was not choosing to be disruptive. His nervous system was responding to an environment that felt threatening, and the school was responding to his survival responses with punishment. The cycle would not change until the approach changed.

Trauma Informed Schools

A growing number of schools are adopting what is called a **trauma informed approach**, which means the school operates with an understanding that many students have experienced adversity and that behavior often communicates unmet needs. In a trauma informed school, discipline focuses on teaching rather than punishing. Staff are trained to recognize trauma responses. And the environment is intentionally designed to reduce triggers (Cole et al., 2005).

If your child's school uses a trauma informed framework, you have a head start. If it does not (and most schools do not yet), you will need to educate the staff yourself, which is frustrating but possible.

The starting point is a conversation with your child's teacher and the school counselor. You do not need to share your child's full trauma history. You need to share what helps and what does not. "My child does best with predictable routines and advance notice of changes." "Raised voices are very activating for my child." "When my child shuts down, it is not defiance; it is a stress response, and they need a few quiet minutes to recover." These are practical, actionable pieces of information that a teacher can use without knowing the underlying story.

IEPs and 504 Plans

Two federal laws provide frameworks for getting your child educational support: the Individuals with Disabilities Education Act (IDEA) and Section 504 of the Rehabilitation Act.

An **IEP** (Individualized Education Program) is available under IDEA for students who have a disability that affects their educational performance. CPTSD can qualify a child for an IEP under the category of "Emotional Disturbance" or, in some cases, "Other Health Impairment." An IEP provides specialized instruction, related services (such as counseling or occupational therapy), and measurable annual goals. It is a legally binding document, and the school is required to provide the services listed in it.

A **504 Plan** is available under Section 504 for students who have a disability that substantially limits one or more major life activities (including learning). A 504 Plan provides accommodations within the general education setting but does not include specialized instruction or the same level of procedural protections as an IEP. However, it is often easier to obtain and can be effective for children whose primary needs are environmental adjustments rather than modified curriculum (Wright & Wright, 2007).

To request either an IEP evaluation or a 504 Plan, put your request in writing. Send a letter or email to the school principal and the director of special education. State that you are requesting an evaluation under IDEA (for an IEP) or accommodations under Section 504. Describe the specific ways your child's functioning is affected at school. The school is required to respond within a specified timeline (which varies by state) and cannot refuse to evaluate without providing a written explanation.

Accommodations That Work

Not all accommodations are equally helpful for children with CPTSD. Generic accommodations (extra time on tests, preferential seating) may not address the actual needs. Here are accommodations that target the specific challenges of complex trauma.

A planned safe space the child can access independently when they feel overwhelmed (a calm corner, the counselor's office, a designated room). This is not a reward or a punishment. It is a regulation tool, similar to the safe spaces described in Chapter 6.0.

A trusted adult the child can go to when dysregulated. This person should be identified in advance and available consistently. For some children, the relationship with one reliable adult at school makes the difference between managing and falling apart.

Advance notice of changes to routine (substitute teachers, fire drills, schedule alterations). For children whose nervous systems depend on predictability, unannounced changes can trigger meltdowns that derail the entire day.

Modified discipline responses. Instead of suspension for behavior that stems from a trauma response, the child receives a structured de-escalation protocol, a restorative conversation, or a shortened day. Zero tolerance policies are particularly harmful for traumatized children because they treat survival behavior as willful misconduct.

Sensory accommodations: permission to use noise canceling headphones, fidget tools, or a weighted lap pad. Permission to take movement breaks. Reduced exposure to chaotic environments (eating lunch in a quieter space, using a hallway pass to avoid crowded transitions).

Reduced homework expectations during periods of high stress. Trauma flares can make home a space where the child is already using all their regulatory capacity, and adding academic demands on top of that can increase family conflict without producing educational benefit.

Check in and check out systems. The child meets briefly with a trusted adult at the beginning and end of each school day. This provides a relational anchor and helps the adult gauge the child's regulatory state before academic demands begin.

When the School Punishes Instead of Supports

Consider Merrick (name changed), the eight year old from Chapter 5.0 whose three day suspension for hitting confirmed his belief that every place would eventually reject him. Merrick's grandmother challenged the suspension through the school's discipline review process, arguing that the behavior was a manifestation of his disability. Under IDEA, if a child's behavior is determined to be a manifestation of their disability, the school cannot suspend them for more than 10 days without providing alternative services.

This process, called a **manifestation determination review** (MDR), is a critical protection for children with IEPs. If your child is facing suspension or expulsion and has an IEP, request an MDR in writing. The school team must determine whether the behavior was caused by or substantially related to the child's disability. If it was, the child cannot be removed from their placement without a plan to address the behavior through the IEP.

If your child does not have an IEP, the school is not required to conduct an MDR. This is one of the strongest reasons to pursue an IEP rather than (or in addition to) a 504 Plan for a child whose trauma related behavior puts them at risk of disciplinary exclusion.

Communicating Without Oversharing

You may feel pressure to tell the school everything about your child's trauma history in order to get them the help they need. Resist this pressure. The school needs to know what your child needs, not every detail of what happened to them.

A framework that works: "My child has experienced significant early adversity that affects their ability to regulate emotions, manage transitions, and respond to authority figures. Here is what helps. Here is what does not help. Here is what their therapist recommends for the school setting."

You can provide a letter from your child's therapist that explains the child's functional limitations and recommended accommodations without disclosing the specific nature of the trauma. This protects your child's privacy while giving the school the information it needs to act.

Consider Crispin (name changed), the 12 year old from Chapter 2.0. His foster parents provided the school with a one page letter from his therapist that described his difficulty with transitions, his need for predictability, and his tendency to shut down when he felt threatened. The letter did not mention his specific trauma history. It gave the school enough to create an effective 504 Plan without exposing Crispin's story to every staff member in the building.

Alternative Schooling Options

For some children with CPTSD, the traditional school environment is simply too activating, even with accommodations. If your child is in crisis at school more often than they are learning, it may be time to consider alternatives.

Therapeutic day schools are designed for children with significant emotional and behavioral needs. Class sizes are small, staff are trained in trauma, and therapeutic support is built into the school day. These placements can be funded through the IEP process if the school district determines that the child cannot make adequate progress in a less restrictive setting.

Homeschooling or virtual schooling provides maximum control over the environment and pacing. For children who need a period of stability and decompression before re-entering a group setting, home based education can be a bridge.

Hybrid models combine some in person instruction with some home based learning. This can work well for children who benefit from social contact but cannot sustain a full school day.

Consider Oswin (name changed), the 14 year old from Chapter 5.0. After two years of escalating behavioral incidents at his traditional school, his foster parents and treatment team agreed that the environment was doing more harm than good. His IEP team placed him in a therapeutic day program where the class size was eight students and every staff member was trained in trauma informed de-escalation. Within one semester, Oswin's behavioral incidents dropped from weekly to monthly. "He didn't become a different kid," his foster mother said. "The school became a different school."

Bringing It Forward

Advocating for your child at school is exhausting, often adversarial, and deeply important. The school environment can either support your child's healing or undermine it, and you are the person who ensures it does the former. You do not need to be a special education attorney. You need to know your child's rights, communicate clearly, and document everything.

In Chapter 14.0, we turn inward, to the rest of your family. The siblings who are affected, the co-parenting relationship that is strained, and the extended family members who may not understand what you are living through.

Chapter 14.0 The Rest of the Family

CPTSD does not affect only the child who has it. It reshapes the entire family system. Siblings grow up in the wake of crisis. Partners disagree about how to respond. Grandparents offer advice that does not apply. And the household operates at a level of intensity that would be unsustainable for anyone, yet somehow you sustain it.

This chapter addresses the family members who orbit around the child with CPTSD. It is about protecting siblings, aligning with co-parents, educating extended family, and recognizing when the strain on your relationship needs attention of its own.

Siblings in the Wake

If you have other children in the home, they are being affected by what is happening, even if they do not show it in obvious ways. Living with a sibling who has severe emotional dysregulation means living with uncertainty, disrupted routines, and a disproportionate share of parental attention directed at the child in crisis.

Siblings of children with CPTSD may experience **secondary traumatic stress**, which means they develop their own anxiety, hypervigilance, or emotional dysregulation from repeated exposure to their sibling's crises. They may also develop feelings of resentment, guilt, invisibility, or fear (Feinberg et al., 2012).

Some siblings become parentified, taking on caregiving roles that are not appropriate for their age. They may try to calm the sibling in crisis, protect younger children, or manage the household emotional temperature. Others withdraw, becoming very quiet and "easy" because they have learned that the family cannot handle another source of difficulty. Both patterns represent children who are adapting to an environment of chronic stress, and both deserve attention.

Consider Larkin (name changed), the 10 year old from Chapter 5.0. His adoptive parents also had a seven year old biological daughter. For the first year after Larkin's placement, their daughter was cooperative and uncomplaining. She never objected when plans were canceled because of Larkin's meltdowns. She never said she was upset when her birthday party was interrupted by a crisis. Then, one evening at dinner, she said quietly, "I wish I was the one who was sick, because then you would pay attention to me." Her parents were devastated. They had been so focused on Larkin's needs that they had not seen what was happening to their daughter.

Talking to Siblings

Children deserve age appropriate honesty about what is happening in their family. They do not need clinical terminology. They need language that validates their experience and gives them a framework for understanding their sibling's behavior.

For young children (ages four to seven): "Your brother's brain got hurt before he came to live with us, and sometimes his feelings get really big and scary for him. When that happens, we need to help him feel safe. That is not your job. Your job is to be a kid. And I always have time for you, even when things are loud."

For school age children (ages eight to 12): "Your sister experienced some really hard things before she was part of our family, and those experiences changed the way her brain handles stress. That's why she sometimes acts the way she does. It's not your fault. It's not her fault. Our family is working on helping her heal, and I know it's hard on you too. I want to hear about how you're doing."

For teenagers: "What's happening with your sibling is real and it's hard. You might feel angry, scared, embarrassed, or resentful, and all of those feelings are valid. You are not responsible for fixing this. You are allowed to need things too. And I want to make sure you have someone to talk to about how this affects you."

Every conversation should include two messages: this is not your fault, and your feelings matter too.

Protecting One on One Time

One of the most effective things you can do for your other children is to protect regular, predictable time that belongs only to them. This does not have to be elaborate. Twenty minutes of undivided attention, doing something the child chooses, on a predictable schedule, can communicate more than any conversation about how much they matter.

The key is consistency. If you schedule Saturday morning breakfast with your daughter, keep it. If a crisis with the other child interrupts, acknowledge the interruption honestly ("I'm sorry our time got cut short. That wasn't fair to you. Let's reschedule for this afternoon.") and follow through. Every kept commitment teaches the sibling that they are not an afterthought.

Consider Fenwick (name changed), the eight year old from Chapter 3.0. His adoptive parents also had a 12 year old son. After noticing that the older boy had become increasingly withdrawn, they implemented a weekly "brother night" with the father: a standing Tuesday evening activity, just the two of them, that happened regardless of what else was occurring in the household. The older boy began talking more openly during those evenings, and his withdrawal decreased. "He just needed to know he had a space that was his," his father said.

Co-Parenting Alignment

If you are parenting with a partner, CPTSD will test your alignment in ways you may not have anticipated. One parent may lean toward the trauma informed approach described in this book while the other maintains that traditional discipline is what the child needs. One parent may feel more patience while the other is burning out faster. One may handle the daily crises while the other handles logistics, creating an imbalance that builds resentment over time.

The most important thing you can do as co-parents is get on the same page about what is happening with your child. Share this book. Attend therapy sessions together when possible. Discuss your approach regularly, not during a crisis, but during calm moments when you can think clearly.

When disagreements arise (and they will), try to keep two principles in front of you. First, disagree in private and present a consistent approach to the child. Children with CPTSD are highly attuned to conflict between caregivers, because caregiver conflict was often a feature of their traumatic environment. Visible disagreement about how to handle the child can activate their alarm system and undermine the felt safety you are trying to build. Second, assume good intent. Your partner is not trying to harm the child by using a different approach. They are likely operating from their own upbringing, their own stress, and their own understanding. The conversation needs to be collaborative, not accusatory.

If one parent is further along in understanding trauma informed parenting, patience with the other parent matters. Just as your child's brain needs time to rewire, your partner may need time to shift their framework. Sending articles, sharing podcast episodes, or inviting them to a parent support group can be more effective than arguing during a meltdown.

If co-parenting alignment feels impossible, consider working with a family therapist who specializes in adoptive, foster, or kinship families. This is not a sign of failure. It is a recognition that parenting a traumatized child places extraordinary demands

on a partnership, and those demands deserve professional
support.

Educating Extended Family

Grandparents, aunts, uncles, and family friends often have strong
opinions about your child's behavior and your response to it.
Many of those opinions come from a place of genuine concern.
And many of them are wrong.

"You just need to be firmer." "That child needs a good
consequence." "In my day, kids didn't act like that because we
didn't allow it." "You're coddling them." "If you just gave them a
good spanking, this would stop."

These comments are painful because they imply that the problem
is your parenting, when in reality the problem is your child's
neurological response to trauma. They are also dangerous,
because if you internalize them, you may return to the very
approaches this book explains will not work (Chapter 5.0).

You have three options with extended family: educate, set
boundaries, or limit contact. The choice depends on the person
and their willingness to learn.

For family members who are willing to learn, offer a simple
explanation: "Our child's brain was affected by what happened to
them before they were with us. The behaviors you're seeing are
not discipline problems. They're stress responses. The strategies
that work for other kids don't work for ours, and our therapist has
given us a different approach." You can share specific chapters of
this book, recommend a shorter resource, or invite them to a
therapy session if the therapist is willing.

For family members who dismiss or undermine your approach,
set boundaries. "I understand you see it differently. We're
following the guidance of our child's treatment team, and I need
you to respect that when you're in our home." You do not owe

anyone an argument. You owe your child a consistent environment.

Consider Quinlan (name changed), the foster father from Chapter 6.0. His mother repeatedly criticized his use of PACE with his foster son, telling him he was "rewarding bad behavior." After several conversations that went nowhere, Quinlan said, "Mom, I love you, and I need you to trust me on this. I'm following what the professionals have told us to do. If you can't support that when you're here, I need you to visit less often." The conversation was difficult. But his mother, after some initial hurt, began asking questions instead of giving advice. "She didn't change overnight," Quinlan said. "But she stopped working against us."

Recognizing Strain on Your Partnership

The divorce and separation rate among parents of children with significant behavioral or emotional challenges is higher than the general population, and CPTSD adds layers of stress that can be particularly corrosive. Sleep deprivation, constant crisis management, reduced social life, financial strain from therapy and medical costs, and the emotional weight of absorbing your child's pain all take a toll on your relationship with your partner (Hartley et al., 2010).

Warning signs include persistent conflict about the child that never resolves, one partner disengaging from parenting responsibilities, loss of physical or emotional intimacy, one or both partners feeling more like crisis managers than life partners, and resentment that builds silently until it erupts.

If you recognize these signs, treat them as seriously as you would treat a symptom in your child. Seek couples therapy with a clinician who understands the context of parenting a traumatized child. Protect time together that has nothing to do with parenting (even 30 minutes after bedtime). And talk about how you are doing, not just how the child is doing.

Chapter 16.0 addresses your individual wellbeing in more depth. But the health of your partnership is a component of your child's healing environment, because a stable caregiver system is the foundation of felt safety (Chapter 6.0).

Holding It All

Your family is carrying something heavy. Every member is affected, and every member deserves attention. The child with CPTSD needs your primary focus, but the siblings need to be seen, the partnership needs to be tended, and the extended family needs to be managed. This is more than any one person should have to do alone, which is why Chapter 17.0 is about building the village that holds you up.

In Chapter 15.0, we step outside the family and into the systems that your family must navigate: child welfare, courts, insurance, and the bureaucratic structures that can either help or harm.

Chapter 15.0 Navigating Systems

Raising a child with Complex PTSD means more than parenting. It often means navigating institutional systems that were designed for efficiency, not for the specific needs of traumatized children and their families. Child welfare agencies, family courts, insurance companies, school districts, and government benefit programs all play a role in your family's life, and each one operates with its own rules, timelines, and priorities.

This chapter is a practical guide to surviving those systems without being consumed by them. It addresses the most common institutional encounters families face, the rights you have within each system, and the documentation practices that protect your child and your family.

Child Welfare and CPS

If your child entered your family through the child welfare system, you are already familiar with the bureaucratic weight of child protective services (CPS). If you are a biological parent whose child was involved with CPS due to circumstances in the home, you may carry additional complexity and grief around that history. And if you are a kinship caregiver who stepped in during a family crisis, you may be navigating CPS while also processing your own feelings about what happened to a child you love within your own family.

Regardless of your entry point, there are several things to know.

You have the right to access your child's case file, including documentation of their placement history, services provided, and any assessments completed while they were in state custody. This information can be critical for your child's current treatment providers, who need a complete picture to make accurate diagnoses and develop effective treatment plans.

You have the right to participate in case planning meetings and to advocate for services your child needs, including trauma focused therapy, psychiatric evaluation, and educational support. If you are a foster or kinship caregiver, you are legally entitled to be heard at every court review and planning meeting.

You have the right to challenge decisions that you believe are not in your child's best interest. If a caseworker recommends reducing therapy services, changing placement, or reunifying the child with a parent who has not completed a safety plan, you can request a review, consult an attorney, or contact your state's foster parent ombudsman.

Consider Bramwell (name changed), the kinship caregiver from Chapter 1.0. When his niece's case moved toward reunification with her mother, Bramwell was concerned because the mother had not yet completed the substance use treatment required by the case plan. He requested a meeting with the caseworker, submitted a written summary of his concerns, and asked for an independent evaluation of the mother's readiness. The court delayed reunification by three months, during which the mother completed treatment. "I wasn't trying to keep her from her mother," Bramwell said. "I was trying to make sure the transition was safe."

Court Involved Families

If your family is involved in family court (whether through custody disputes, adoption proceedings, dependency hearings, or juvenile justice matters), the court system will make decisions that profoundly affect your child's life. Courts are not therapeutic environments. They are adversarial by design, and the needs of a traumatized child can get lost in legal proceedings.

Here are some practical recommendations.

Request that any court ordered evaluations be conducted by professionals with training in developmental trauma. A standard custody evaluation or psychological assessment that does not account for CPTSD may produce misleading conclusions (for example, interpreting the child's attachment behavior as evidence of one parent's influence rather than as a trauma response).

If your child must testify or participate in a court process, request accommodations: a support person present, closed circuit testimony, or a written statement in lieu of in person testimony. Court appearances are stressful for any child. For a traumatized child, they can be retraumatizing.

Document everything. Keep copies of all court orders, correspondence with attorneys, and reports from evaluators. Maintain a log of your child's behavior, therapy progress, and any incidents that are relevant to the court proceedings. This documentation can make the difference between a decision made on assumptions and a decision made on evidence.

If you cannot afford an attorney, contact your local legal aid society. Many jurisdictions have attorneys who specialize in representing foster parents, kinship caregivers, or parents in dependency proceedings at reduced or no cost.

Insurance Battles

Getting insurance to cover appropriate treatment for childhood CPTSD is one of the most frustrating experiences families face. Here is why it is difficult and what you can do.

Many insurance plans cover a limited number of therapy sessions per year, which is inadequate for the long term treatment that CPTSD requires. Many plans do not cover specific modalities (such as EMDR or neurofeedback) or restrict coverage to providers who are in network (where trauma specialists may be scarce). And because CPTSD is not in the DSM-5, some insurers may deny coverage for treatments specifically targeting complex trauma, arguing that the diagnosis is not recognized.

Strategies for navigating these barriers include the following. Ask your child's therapist to use DSM-5 codes that the insurer will recognize (such as PTSD, generalized anxiety disorder, or adjustment disorder with mixed disturbance of emotions and conduct) while still delivering trauma focused treatment. This is not dishonest. It is a practical response to a system that has not caught up with the clinical reality.

If a claim is denied, appeal. Most denials are overturned on appeal, but most families never appeal because the process seems overwhelming. Your child's therapist or psychiatrist can write a letter of medical necessity explaining why the specific treatment is required for your child's condition. Many states have independent review processes for denied mental health claims.

If your child is on Medicaid, research your state's specific coverage for children's mental health services. Many states have Medicaid waivers or special programs that provide enhanced coverage for children with significant behavioral health needs, including therapeutic foster care, intensive in home services, and residential treatment when necessary.

Consider Jory (name changed), the 13 year old from Chapter 4.0. His family's private insurance initially denied coverage for EMDR, stating it was "experimental." His therapist submitted a letter of medical necessity citing the published evidence base for EMDR in the treatment of PTSD, along with documentation of Jory's treatment history and lack of progress with other approaches. The denial was reversed on appeal. "I nearly gave up after the first denial," his mother said. "I'm glad I didn't."

Adoption Subsidies and Respite Care

If your child was adopted from foster care, you may be eligible for an adoption subsidy (sometimes called adoption assistance). These subsidies are designed to help offset the costs of raising a child with special needs and can cover therapy copays, medical expenses, and other costs. The terms of the subsidy are negotiated at the time of adoption, but they can often be renegotiated if the child's needs change.

Respite care is another resource that many families underuse. Respite provides temporary relief for caregivers by arranging for the child to spend time with a trained respite provider (usually for a weekend or a few hours). Some states fund respite through the child welfare system, through Medicaid waivers, or through adoption assistance programs. Others have nonprofit organizations that provide respite services.

Consider Kenrick (name changed), the nine year old from Chapter 4.0. His parents negotiated a respite plan as part of his adoption agreement: one weekend per month with a trained respite provider who was familiar with Kenrick's needs. "At first I felt guilty," his mother said. "Like I was sending him away. But our therapist helped me see that respite isn't abandonment. It's sustainability. I can't help him if I'm burned out."

Respite is not a luxury. It is a clinical recommendation for families raising children with significant trauma histories. We discuss this further in Chapter 17.0.

Building Your Documentation Habit

If you take one practical step from this chapter, let it be this: document everything. Every phone call with a caseworker, every school meeting, every insurance denial, every therapy recommendation. Keep a running log with dates, the names of the people you spoke with, and what was discussed or decided.

This documentation serves multiple purposes. It creates a record you can reference when your memory is unreliable (which it will be, because chronic stress impairs memory). It provides evidence when you need to appeal a decision, challenge a disciplinary action, or demonstrate your child's needs in court. And it gives you a sense of agency in systems that often make parents feel powerless.

A simple notebook or a notes app on your phone is sufficient. Date each entry. Note who you talked to and what was said. Save copies of important documents (IEPs, court orders, insurance correspondence, therapy reports) in a folder, physical or digital, that you can access quickly.

When communicating with any system, follow up verbal conversations with written confirmation. After a phone call with a caseworker, send an email: "Thank you for our conversation today. To confirm, we discussed [topic] and the next step is [action] by [date]. Please let me know if I have captured this incorrectly." This creates a paper trail that protects you if the system later claims something different was agreed upon.

When attending meetings (IEP meetings, case planning conferences, court hearings), bring your documentation folder. Having dates, names, and prior agreements at your fingertips communicates that you are organized and informed, which changes how systems treat you. It also prevents the common experience of being told, "We never agreed to that," when you know you did.

Institutional Retraumatization

A painful reality that must be named: the systems designed to help your child can also harm your child. Every time your child is required to retell their trauma story to a new evaluator, caseworker, or judge, they are re-exposed to that story. Every time they are moved between placements, they lose the relational continuity their nervous system depends on. Every time they are subjected to punitive discipline for trauma related behavior, the institution confirms what the child already believes: that they are too much, too damaged, and unworthy of patient, informed care.

This is called **institutional retraumatization**, and it is one of the most significant obstacles to healing for children in systems (Substance Abuse and Mental Health Services Administration, 2014).

You cannot single handedly reform these systems. But you can minimize their harm by controlling what you can control. Limit the number of times your child must tell their story. Provide written summaries to new providers instead of requiring the child to recount events in person. Challenge disciplinary practices that punish trauma responses. And when you see a system failing your child, name it (in writing, to the relevant authorities, with documentation) so that the failure is on the record.

Consider Dunstan (name changed), the 15 year old from Chapter 2.0. Over the course of his involvement with the juvenile justice system (following the stealing incident), he was required to tell his history to four different evaluators, two judges, and three caseworkers. Each retelling activated his trauma response. His mother began requesting that existing evaluations be shared between providers rather than conducting new ones. "I told them: you have his story. It's in the file. Stop making him relive it for your paperwork."

Getting Through

The systems you navigate are imperfect. They are underfunded, understaffed, and frequently organized around bureaucratic convenience rather than the needs of traumatized children. Working within them is exhausting. But understanding your rights, documenting your interactions, and advocating persistently can shift outcomes in your child's favor.

In Part Five, we turn to the person who has been holding all of this together: you. Chapters 16.0 through 18.0 address your own trauma responses, your need for support, and the long view of what healing looks like for your family.

Part Five: Sustaining Yourself

Caregiver Health, Hope, and the Long Road

Chapter 16.0 The Parent Behind the Parent

Every chapter in this book so far has been about your child. This one is about you.

Not about you as a caregiver, a case manager, an advocate, or a crisis responder. About you as a person who is being changed by this experience in ways you may not have had time to examine. Because when you parent a child with Complex PTSD, the child's pain does not stay neatly contained within the child. It reaches into you. It activates things you thought you had settled. It exhausts resources you did not know were finite. And if no one tells you that this is happening and that it is normal, you may begin to believe that the problem is you.

It is not you. But it does need your attention.

Why This Work Activates Your Own Wounds

Parenting a traumatized child involves daily exposure to distress, dysregulation, rejection, and fear. Even if you have no trauma history of your own, this exposure affects you. And if you do carry your own history of adverse experiences (which a significant number of foster, adoptive, and kinship parents do), parenting a child with CPTSD can reactivate neural pathways you may have spent years learning to manage (Figley, 2002).

This happens because of the same mirror neuron system and co-regulation dynamics described in Chapter 7.0. When your child is in distress, your nervous system responds. Your heart rate increases. Your muscles tense. Your breathing changes. If your child screams "I hate you," your body does not process that statement as clinical data. It processes it as a relational injury. And if your own childhood included moments when the people who were supposed to love you said similar things, or worse, the old wound opens alongside the new one.

This is not weakness. It is neurobiology. Your brain is doing exactly what brains do: recognizing a pattern and responding to it based on prior experience. The problem is that when your own stress response is activated at the same time as your child's, your capacity to co-regulate (the very thing your child needs most) is compromised. You cannot lend calm if you have none to spare.

Consider Elowen (name changed), the foster mother from Chapter 1.0. She described a moment when her daughter screamed, "You're not my real mom! I want my real mom!" Elowen's conscious mind knew this was a trauma response. Her body did not care. She felt her chest tighten, her eyes burn, and a wave of shame rise from somewhere deep. Later, in her own therapy, she traced the reaction to her childhood experience of being told by her mother that she was "too much." Her daughter's words had activated a wound that predated the foster placement by 30 years.

Elowen's experience illustrates something important: you do not need to have experienced the same kind of trauma as your child for your own history to be activated. What matters is whether the emotional tone of the current moment resembles something your nervous system has filed as threatening.

Knowing Your Triggers

Just as Chapter 8.0 helped you map your child's triggers, this section asks you to map your own. Your triggers as a parent are the moments when your response is disproportionate to the situation, when you feel flooded, when you shut down, or when you react in ways you later regret. These moments are data, not failures.

Common parental triggers when raising a child with CPTSD include the following. Being rejected by the child you are trying

to help. Feeling helpless when nothing you do seems to work.
Being hit, kicked, or physically threatened. Hearing the child use
language that mirrors something from your own past. Witnessing
the child's pain and being unable to take it away. Being judged by
others (schools, family members, strangers) for your child's
behavior. Having your authority challenged repeatedly. Feeling
invisible as a person because you have become nothing but a
caregiver.

Take a moment to identify which of these resonate for you. There
may be others not listed. The goal is not to eliminate your
triggers (that is not possible) but to recognize them, so that when
they fire, you have a fraction of a second to choose your response
rather than being carried by the reaction.

Consider Bramwell (name changed), the kinship caregiver from
Chapter 1.0. He noticed that his most intense reactions happened
when his niece refused to eat the meals he prepared. On the
surface, this seemed like a minor issue. But when he explored it
in therapy, he connected the refusal to his own childhood
experience of food scarcity. His niece's rejection of food felt, to
his nervous system, like a rejection of the safety he was trying to
provide. Once he named the trigger, he could catch it. "When she
pushes the plate away, I remind myself: this is her nervous
system, not mine. Her refusal is not my failure."

Secondary Traumatic Stress and Compassion Fatigue

Secondary traumatic stress (STS) is a clinical term for the
impact of repeated exposure to another person's trauma. It can
produce symptoms that mirror PTSD itself: intrusive thoughts
about the child's history, hypervigilance, sleep disruption,
emotional numbing, irritability, and a persistent sense of dread.
STS is well documented in professionals who work with
traumatized populations (therapists, social workers, first
responders), but it is less often discussed in the context of
parents, even though parents have far more sustained exposure
than any professional (Figley, 2002).

Compassion fatigue is related but distinct. It describes the gradual erosion of your capacity to care. You may notice that you feel less empathy than you used to. That your child's distress, which once moved you deeply, now produces irritation or blankness. That you go through the motions of caregiving without feeling connected to the child or to yourself. Compassion fatigue is not a character flaw. It is the predictable result of sustained emotional output without adequate replenishment (Stamm, 2010).

If you recognize yourself in either of these descriptions, please hear this clearly: this does not mean you are failing as a parent. It means you are a human being who has been operating under extraordinary stress for an extended period, and your system is telling you it needs help.

Signs that you may be experiencing STS or compassion fatigue include persistent sleep problems not explained by other causes, emotional numbness or feeling disconnected from your own life, increased irritability or anger that is out of proportion to the situation, difficulty concentrating or making decisions, physical symptoms such as chronic headaches, stomach problems, or fatigue, withdrawal from friends, activities, or your partner, feeling trapped or hopeless about the parenting situation, and intrusive images or thoughts related to your child's trauma history.

Getting Your Own Therapy

If your child has a therapist, you need access to support too. This may be individual therapy, a support group, or both. What it should not be is nothing.

Your therapy does not need to be the same modality as your child's. What it needs to be is a space where you can process the emotional impact of what you are living through without worrying about how it affects anyone else. A space where you can say, "I love this child and sometimes I don't like them," without being judged. A space where you can examine your own triggers, grieve the parenting experience you expected, and rebuild the internal resources that daily crisis management depletes.

If you have your own trauma history, therapy is especially important. Parenting a child with CPTSD can surface material you thought was resolved. A therapist trained in trauma (using the same criteria described in Chapter 10.0) can help you process that material so that it stops hijacking your parenting responses.

Consider Crispin (name changed), the 12 year old from Chapter 2.0. His foster father, who had grown up in a household with an alcoholic parent, began having nightmares after Crispin moved in. The nightmares were not about Crispin. They were about his own childhood. "Parenting him opened a door I thought I had closed," he said. He started seeing a therapist who specialized in adult survivors of childhood adversity, and the nightmares reduced within two months. "I can't help him heal from trauma if I'm drowning in my own," he said. He was right.

Body Based Regulation for Parents

The same nervous system principles that apply to your child apply to you. When you are dysregulated, your thinking brain goes offline and your survival brain takes over. You cannot co-regulate from that state. So building your own regulation capacity is not self indulgence. It is a parenting strategy.

Here are body based practices that research supports for reducing physiological activation in caregivers.

Slow breathing. Inhale for four counts, hold for four, exhale for six to eight. The extended exhale activates the parasympathetic nervous system and sends a signal of safety to the brain. Practice this when you are calm so that it becomes accessible when you are not (Porges, 2011).

Progressive muscle tension and release. Starting with your feet and moving upward, tense each muscle group for five seconds, then release. This helps discharge the physical tension that accumulates during sustained stress.

Cold water. Splashing cold water on your face or holding an ice cube activates the dive reflex, which slows heart rate and reduces sympathetic activation. This can be useful in the moments immediately after a crisis when your body is still buzzing.

Movement. Walking, stretching, dancing, or any physical activity that moves your body out of the frozen or clenched state that chronic stress produces. Even five minutes can shift your nervous system state.

These are not replacements for therapy or community support. They are immediate, accessible tools for the moments when you need to reclaim your calm before you can give it to your child.

Permission to Grieve

Chapter 5.0 introduced the concept of grieving the parenting experience you expected. This chapter returns to it because grief does not appear once and resolve. It cycles. You may grieve when you see other families at the park, functioning with an ease you cannot remember. You may grieve on your child's birthday, thinking about the milestones that trauma delayed. You may grieve at the end of a day that was consumed by crisis management, with no space left for joy, play, or rest.

This grief is real. It deserves to be named, felt, and held, not pushed aside because "other people have it worse" or because naming your pain feels like a betrayal of your child. You can love your child fiercely and still grieve what this experience has cost you. Those two truths coexist.

Consider Kenrick (name changed), the nine year old from Chapter 4.0. His mother described a moment at a family gathering where she watched her sister's children playing calmly while Kenrick hid under a table, refusing to come out. "I felt this wave of sadness that I couldn't explain to anyone in the room," she said. "Not sadness for him. Sadness for the version of motherhood I thought I would have. And then guilt for feeling sad, because he is the one who suffered." Her therapist helped her see that the grief and the love were not in competition. Both were true. Both needed space.

What This Costs and What It Gives

Parenting a child with CPTSD will change you. It will cost you sleep, friendships, peace of mind, and parts of the life you planned. But it will also teach you things about yourself that you could not have learned any other way. It will show you how deep your capacity for patience actually runs. It will teach you to sit with pain without trying to fix it, a skill that will serve every relationship you have for the rest of your life. And on the days when your child takes a step forward, however small, you will feel a kind of joy that people who have never walked this road cannot fully understand.

In Chapter 17.0, we address the support system you need around you to sustain this work. You were never meant to do it alone.

Chapter 17.0 Building Your Village

The most consistent finding in the research on caregiver wellbeing is also the most intuitive: parents who have support do better, and their children do better as a result. The inverse is equally true. Isolation is one of the most damaging forces in the life of a family raising a child with CPTSD. When you are alone with the daily weight of crisis, advocacy, and grief, the weight does not lighten. It compounds (Purvis et al., 2013).

This chapter is about building the network of people, organizations, and resources that can hold you up when you cannot hold yourself. It is also about the practical reality that asking for help is difficult, that friendships change when your life looks nothing like your friends' lives, and that the village you need may not assemble itself. You may have to build it.

Finding Your People

The most powerful source of support for parents raising traumatized children is other parents who are doing the same thing. Not because they have all the answers, but because they understand the questions. They know what it is like to explain to a teacher that your child's behavior is not a discipline problem. They know the particular exhaustion of a Tuesday morning after a night of screaming. They know the mix of love and frustration that no one outside this experience can fully grasp.

Support groups for parents of traumatized children exist in several forms. In person groups may be offered through your child's therapy practice, your local foster care agency, or community mental health organizations. The National Child Traumatic Stress Network (NCTSN) maintains a directory of programs that include parent support components. Adoptive and foster parent associations in most states run regional support groups, some specifically for families dealing with trauma and attachment difficulties.

Online communities have expanded access significantly. Facebook groups, forums, and moderated online support spaces allow parents in rural or underserved areas to connect with others who share their experience. Some of these groups are moderated by clinicians. Others are peer led. The quality varies, but the principle is consistent: being in a room (physical or virtual) with people who understand your life reduces the isolation that makes everything harder.

Consider Oswin (name changed), the 14 year old from Chapter 5.0. His foster mother described joining an online support group for foster parents of teens with trauma histories. "The first time I posted about a meltdown, and three people responded with 'That happened to us last week,' I cried. Not because they had solutions. Because they knew."

Respite Care

Respite care, introduced in Chapter 15.0, deserves further attention here because it is one of the most underused and most needed resources available to families raising children with CPTSD. Respite means arranging for your child to spend time with a trained caregiver so that you can rest, recover, and attend to the other parts of your life that have been neglected.

Many parents resist respite because it feels like giving up, like admitting that they cannot handle what they signed up for. But respite is not failure. It is maintenance. It is the recognition that a caregiver who is chronically depleted cannot provide the attuned, regulated presence their child needs.

Sources of respite include your state's foster care or adoption support programs (many fund respite directly), Medicaid waiver programs that include respite hours, nonprofit organizations such as the ARCH National Respite Network, and informal arrangements with trained and trusted adults in your community.

If formal respite is not available, informal respite matters too. A family member who takes your other children for an afternoon. A friend who brings dinner so you do not have to cook. A neighbor who sits in the driveway (available by text) while you take a bath. These small acts of support accumulate, and they are worth asking for.

Consider Aldwyn (name changed), the nine year old from Chapter 2.0. His parents arranged for a trained respite provider to spend one Saturday per month with Aldwyn. They used the time for activities they had stopped doing: a long walk, lunch at a restaurant, an hour of uninterrupted conversation. "We came back better every time," his mother said. "Not because we didn't miss him. Because we had something left to give when we walked through the door."

Building a Network of Safe Adults

Your child needs more than one safe adult in their life. You need more than one person who understands your child's needs. Building a small network of informed, reliable people around your family creates resilience for both you and your child.

A safe adult is someone who understands your child's trauma informed needs, who can follow the household approach (connection before correction, predictable routines, PACE), and who your child has had time to build comfort with. This might be a grandparent who has read this book, a close friend who has spent enough time in your home to understand the patterns, a respite provider, or a mentor from your faith community.

Building this network takes intentional effort. It means having honest conversations with the people in your life about what your child needs and what you need. It means educating willing adults about trauma responses (sharing specific chapters, inviting them to a therapy session, providing a one page summary of your child's triggers and de-escalation strategies). And it means accepting that some people in your life will not be able to be part of this network, and that is a loss worth grieving but not a reason to stop building.

Asking for Help

Asking for help is one of the hardest things for caregivers of traumatized children. You may feel that no one can handle your child. You may feel that explaining what you need takes more energy than just doing it yourself. You may have been burned by offers of help that evaporated when the reality became clear. Or you may have internalized the belief that needing help means failing.

Here are scripts for asking, because sometimes having the words ready makes the difference between asking and not asking.

To a friend: "I am going through a really intense time with my child. I don't need you to understand all of it. I need you to check in on me sometimes and not take it personally if I cancel plans. And if you're ever available to bring a meal or sit with my other kids for an hour, that would mean more than you know."

To a family member: "Our family is dealing with something that requires a different approach than what you might expect. I would love for you to be part of our support system. That means trusting our approach even when it looks different from how you would handle it. I can share some resources if you're interested."

To your child's school: "I am requesting a team meeting to discuss how we can better support my child. I want to work collaboratively, and I need the school to be part of the solution."

To your own therapist: "I am noticing that I am running on empty and my reactions are getting bigger. I need help with my own regulation so I can keep showing up for my child."

The common thread in all of these scripts is honesty without apology. You are not asking for a favor. You are identifying what you need in order to sustain the work of raising your child.

When Friendships Change

One of the less discussed losses of parenting a child with CPTSD is the quiet fading of friendships that cannot survive the distance between your experience and theirs. Friends who used to call may call less. Invitations to social events may thin out, partly because you have had to cancel so many times, partly because your life now occupies a space that makes casual socializing difficult.

This is painful. And it does not mean those friends are bad people. It means your lives have diverged, and the gap is hard to bridge from either side. You may find that the friendships that endure are the ones where the other person can tolerate not understanding and stays present anyway. Those friendships are worth protecting.

Some practical ways to maintain friendships during this season: be honest about your capacity ("I can't do dinner out, but I can talk on the phone for 20 minutes after bedtime"). Let people know what kind of support helps ("I don't need advice right now. I need someone to listen."). And give yourself permission to grieve the friendships that fade without turning the grief into guilt.

New friendships may also form, often with other parents in similar situations. These friendships carry a particular intimacy because they are grounded in shared experience. The parent you meet at a support group who texts you at 11 p.m. during a meltdown. The adoptive parent across town who trades respite days with you. These connections may look different from the friendships you had before, but they may also be among the most meaningful of your life.

Consider Merrick (name changed), the eight year old from Chapter 5.0. His grandmother described losing most of her social circle in the first year of caregiving. "My friends didn't know what to say, and I didn't have energy to teach them." But through a local kinship care support group, she met two other grandmothers raising grandchildren with trauma histories. "We text every day. We know each other's children's triggers. We take turns having hard weeks. That group saved me."

Consider Jory (name changed), the 13 year old from Chapter 4.0. His mother, who had been parenting Jory through years of escalating diagnoses and treatment changes, described the turning point: "I was at a conference for parents of kids with trauma, and a woman stood up and described my exact Tuesday. My exact Tuesday. I walked up to her afterward and said, 'Can we be friends?' That was three years ago. She's now the person I call first." The connection was not built on shared hobbies or proximity. It was built on shared understanding. And that understanding, when everything else feels incomprehensible, is its own form of rescue.

Where to Look

The following organizations and resources are starting points for building your support network.

The National Child Traumatic Stress Network (nctsn.org) provides resources for families, a provider directory, and information about evidence based treatments. The ARCH National Respite Network (archrespite.org) helps families locate respite care in their area. The North American Council on Adoptable Children (nacac.org) offers support groups and resources for adoptive families. The National Alliance for Mental Illness (nami.org) provides family support groups and educational programs. Local foster and adoptive parent associations can be found through your state's department of children and family services. The Attachment and Trauma

Network (attachmenttraumanetwork.org) focuses specifically on families raising children with trauma and attachment challenges.

Your child's therapist may also know of local resources, parent mentoring programs, or community organizations that serve families like yours. Ask.

The Village Is Not Optional

This chapter exists because the work you are doing cannot be sustained alone. Not because you are not strong enough. Because no one is. The biological imperative behind co-regulation (Chapter 7.0) applies to you as much as it applies to your child. You need people around you whose calm you can borrow. You need people who can hold part of the weight. You need people who see you, not just as a parent, but as a person.

In Chapter 18.0, we take the longest view. We look at what healing actually looks like over years, what the research says about the capacity of the developing brain to change, and what hope means when you measure it not in days but in decades.

Chapter 18.0 The Long View

This is the last chapter of this book, and it is about something you may have lost sight of along the way: hope. Not the kind of hope that promises everything will be fine. The kind of hope that is grounded in science, sustained by evidence, and available to you and your child even on the hardest days.

Healing from Complex PTSD is not linear. It does not follow a clean upward trajectory. It moves forward and backward and sideways, often in the same week. But it moves. And the fact that your child's brain is still developing means the possibility of change is not just optimistic thinking. It is neurological reality.

The Science of Hope

In Chapter 3.0, we introduced the concept of neuroplasticity: the brain's ability to form new neural pathways in response to new experiences. For children, this capacity is especially strong. The same developmental sensitivity that made your child's brain vulnerable to trauma also makes it responsive to healing. The brain that was shaped by danger can be reshaped by safety, connection, and consistent attuned care (Perry & Szalavitz, 2006).

Research on children who have experienced early adversity and then been placed in stable, responsive environments shows measurable changes in brain structure and function over time. Studies of children adopted from Romanian orphanages into nurturing families found significant recovery in cognitive functioning, emotional regulation, and attachment patterns, particularly when the adoption occurred before age two, but with meaningful gains observed at later ages as well (Rutter et al., 2007).

This does not mean the effects of trauma disappear. Some neural pathways formed during periods of danger will remain. But the brain builds new pathways alongside them, and with enough repetition, the new pathways can become the dominant ones. Your child may always have a sensitive alarm system. But they can learn to manage it. They may always carry the memory of what happened. But they can learn that the memory is the past, not the present.

The critical ingredient in this process, according to the research, is the quality and consistency of the caregiving relationship. Not perfection. Consistency. The parent who shows up, who repairs after ruptures, who regulates themselves enough to help regulate the child, is the most powerful agent of change in the child's life (Baylin & Hughes, 2016).

That parent is you.

What Progress Actually Looks Like

If you are looking for progress in the wrong places, you will miss it. Progress for a child with CPTSD does not look like the sudden absence of symptoms. It looks like subtle shifts that accumulate over months and years.

Progress looks like a meltdown that lasts 20 minutes instead of 90. It looks like the child coming to find you after a rupture instead of hiding for hours. It looks like a single moment of eye contact during a hard conversation. It looks like the child saying "I'm mad" instead of throwing a chair. It looks like sleeping through the night for three nights in a row after months of waking up screaming. It looks like the child asking for help with something small, because asking for help requires trust, and trust is the hardest thing for their brain to build.

Consider Godric (name changed), the 10 year old from Chapter 3.0. After 18 months of trauma therapy, PACE parenting, and a stable home environment, his mother was asked by a friend, "Is he better?" She paused. "He still melts down. He still has nightmares sometimes. He still flinches when someone moves too fast. But last week he told me he was scared. He has never told me he was scared before. He has always just reacted. The fact that he could name it means his thinking brain is coming online. So yes. He's better. It just doesn't look the way people expect."

Why Setbacks Are Not Failures

There will be periods when your child seems to regress. A child who was sleeping well begins having night terrors again. A child who had stopped hoarding food starts again. A teenager who was making progress suddenly blows up and destroys their room. These setbacks can feel devastating, especially after you have worked so hard to create progress.

Setbacks happen for reasons. Anniversaries of traumatic events (even ones the child does not consciously remember) can trigger regression. Developmental transitions (starting a new school year, entering puberty, changing placements) destabilize the nervous system because they introduce unpredictability. Therapy itself, particularly when it moves into the processing phase, can temporarily increase symptoms before they improve.

The setback does not erase the progress. The neural pathways your child has been building do not vanish because of a hard week. They are still there, underneath the current storm. Your job during a setback is not to fix it but to ride it out with your child, using the same tools you have been using all along: felt safety, co-regulation, connection before correction. The storm will pass. The pathways will reassert themselves.

Consider Ivor (name changed), the 11 year old from Chapter 4.0. After a year of trauma focused therapy and consistent parenting, his meltdowns had reduced from daily to weekly. Then his family moved to a new house, and the meltdowns returned to daily. His parents were crushed. But his therapist reminded them: "The move activated his threat system. He's back in survival mode temporarily. But look at what happens during the meltdowns now. He recovers faster. He seeks you out afterward. He says he's sorry. None of that was happening a year ago. The progress isn't gone. It's buried under the stress. When the stress settles, it will be visible again." Six weeks after the move, she was right.

Puberty Through Emerging Adulthood

The transition into adolescence is a challenging period for any child. For a child with CPTSD, puberty introduces a new wave of complexity. Hormonal changes intensify emotions that are already poorly regulated. The developmental drive toward independence conflicts with the child's deep (and often denied) need for dependable caregivers. Social pressures increase. Romantic relationships introduce new triggers around intimacy, trust, and vulnerability. And the adolescent brain's push for autonomy can look, in a child with CPTSD, like a resumption of the rejection and testing behavior that characterized earlier years (Siegel, 2014).

Some specific things to watch for during adolescence. Increased risk taking as the teen's still developing prefrontal cortex and heightened stress response combine to produce impulsive decisions. Substance use as self medication for anxiety, hyperarousal, or emotional pain. Self harm or suicidal ideation, which may increase during periods of intense emotional distress (see Chapter 12.0 for crisis response). Re-emergence of attachment testing, where the teen pushes you away with increasing force to see if you will stay. And identity confusion, as the teen tries to construct a sense of self that incorporates their trauma history without being defined by it.

The parenting principles in this book do not change during adolescence. They adapt. The felt safety strategies become less about sensory environments and more about respecting autonomy. The co-regulation shifts from physical proximity to emotional availability. The scripts become briefer and the silences longer. But the foundation remains: connection, predictability, and the steady message that this relationship is not going away.

The transition from adolescence into young adulthood (ages 18 to 25) brings its own challenges. Your child may age out of systems that provided support (foster care, school accommodations, pediatric mental health services). They may need help navigating adult services, vocational support, or independent living. Many young adults with CPTSD histories experience a period of struggling with independence before finding their footing. Others surprise everyone, including themselves, with resilience that was invisible during the harder years.

Consider Dunstan (name changed), the 15 year old from Chapter 2.0. His mother, speaking three years later, described the arc: "At 15, I thought we were going to lose him. At 17, he started seeing a new therapist and something clicked. At 18, he got a job at a bike shop and started showing up on time. He's not where other 18 year olds are. He's where he needs to be. And that's enough."

The Good Enough Parent

Psychoanalyst Donald Winnicott introduced the concept of the "good enough mother" in the 1950s, and it has never been more relevant than it is for parents of children with CPTSD. Winnicott's point was that children do not need perfect parents. They need parents who are present, responsive, and willing to repair when they fall short (Winnicott, 1971).

You will not get this right every day. You will lose your temper. You will miss cues. You will say the wrong thing, at the wrong time, in the wrong tone. You will have moments where you wonder if you are the right person for this child. And then you will come back. You will repair. You will try again. That pattern, the returning, is what heals.

Consider Quinlan (name changed), the foster father from Chapter 6.0. After a year of raising his foster son, he described his parenting this way: "I thought I had to be perfect. The therapist told me I had to be present. That was different. Perfection is something I can't do. Presence is something I can choose, even when I'm tired, even when I'm angry, even when I don't know what I'm doing. I choose to be here. Every day, I choose to be here."

What Healing Looks Like in the Long Run

Healing from CPTSD is not a destination. It is a direction. Your child may never be entirely free of the effects of what happened to them. But "free of effects" is not the standard. The standard is a life that is not organized around survival. A life where relationships feel more safe than threatening. Where feelings can be named and tolerated. Where the future holds possibility rather than just danger.

Some children who grow up with CPTSD become adults who are remarkably perceptive, compassionate, and resilient, not in spite of what they experienced, but because the work of healing taught them things about themselves and about human connection that most people never learn. This is not a guarantee. It is a possibility that your daily work makes more likely.

Consider Larkin (name changed), the 10 year old from Chapter 5.0. His adoptive mother, looking ahead, said something that captures what the long view feels like from the inside: "I don't know what his life will look like in 20 years. I don't know if he'll go to college or get married or have children of his own. What I know is that every day I show up for him, I am writing a line in a story he doesn't have to carry alone. And I believe, because the science tells me and because I have seen it with my own eyes, that the story is getting better."

A Letter to the Future

If you could write a letter to your child's future self, it might say something like this. You survived something that should not have happened to you. The adults in your early life failed you in ways that changed the shape of your brain and the pattern of your heart. But other adults came along who chose you, who stayed, who learned what you needed and tried their best to provide it. They were not perfect. But they were there. And their presence, day after day, year after year, gave your brain the evidence it needed to update its predictions about the world. You are more than what happened to you. You always were.

And if you could write a letter to your own future self, it might say this. You did something extraordinarily hard. You parented a child the world had already wounded, and you did it with imperfect knowledge, insufficient sleep, and a heart that sometimes felt like it was going to break. You made mistakes. You repaired them. You showed up when every cell in your body wanted to shut down. And the child who once flinched at your touch began, slowly, unevenly, to reach for your hand. That is the evidence. That is the long view. That is enough.

Appendices: Practical Tools,

Resources, and Ready-to-Use Templates

Appendix A: Glossary of Key Terms

The following definitions are written for parents, not clinicians. They describe how each term is used in this book and how it applies to your daily experience with your child.

Amygdala. A small, almond shaped structure deep in the brain that functions as the body's alarm system. It scans the environment for threat and triggers the stress response when danger is detected. In children with CPTSD, the amygdala is overactive, sounding the alarm in response to things that resemble past danger even when the current environment is safe. See Chapter 3.0.

Attachment. The emotional bond between a child and their primary caregiver. Healthy attachment develops when a caregiver is consistently responsive to the child's needs. When early caregiving is harmful, unpredictable, or absent, the child's attachment patterns become insecure or disorganized, affecting how they relate to others throughout life. See Chapters 2.0 and 6.0.

Co-Regulation. The process by which a calm adult helps a dysregulated child return to a regulated state. Before children can manage their own emotions, they need to borrow regulation from an attuned caregiver. Co-regulation happens through tone of voice, facial expression, body language, physical proximity, and steady presence. It is the biological foundation of emotional development. See Chapter 7.0.

Compassion Fatigue. The gradual erosion of a caregiver's capacity to feel empathy and emotional engagement after sustained exposure to another person's suffering. Signs include emotional numbness, irritability, withdrawal, and going through the motions of caregiving without feeling connected. See Chapter 16.0.

Complex Post Traumatic Stress Disorder (CPTSD). A condition that develops after prolonged, repeated exposure to traumatic events, particularly during childhood and involving caregiving relationships. CPTSD includes all the features of PTSD (re-experiencing, avoidance, sense of threat) plus three additional clusters: emotional dysregulation, negative self concept, and disturbed relationships. Included in the ICD-11 but not the DSM-5. See Chapter 2.0.

Developmental Trauma Disorder (DTD). A proposed diagnosis, developed by Bessel van der Kolk and Julian Ford, specifically for children whose complex trauma began early in life and affected their development. DTD captures disrupted attachment, emotional and physical dysregulation, behavioral difficulties, cognitive impairments, and a distorted sense of self. Not yet included in the DSM-5. See Chapter 2.0.

Dissociation. A protective shutdown response in which the mind disconnects from present experience to reduce overwhelming pain. In children, dissociation can look like going blank, staring, not responding to their name, appearing to be "somewhere else," or watching themselves from outside their body. It is a dorsal vagal response (see polyvagal theory below). See Chapters 3.0 and 12.0.

Dorsal Vagal Response. The shutdown or collapse state described in polyvagal theory. When the nervous system determines that neither fighting nor fleeing is possible, it conserves energy by shutting down. Heart rate drops, the child appears flat or unresponsive, and dissociation may occur. See polyvagal theory below and Chapter 3.0.

Emotional Dysregulation. Severe difficulty managing emotional responses. A child with emotional dysregulation may swing rapidly between intense emotions, react with extreme intensity to small provocations, or shut down completely when overwhelmed. It is one of the three core features of CPTSD. See Chapter 2.0.

Emotional Flashback. A re-experiencing of the emotional state associated with a past traumatic event, without a visual memory or conscious awareness that the current feelings are connected to the past. The child (or adult) suddenly feels the terror, shame, helplessness, or rage of the original experience but may not understand why. Emotional flashbacks are driven by implicit memory. See Chapter 3.0.

Explicit Memory. Memories that are consciously accessible and organized with a time stamp and narrative context. You remember what happened, when it happened, and that it is in the past. Contrast with implicit memory. See Chapter 3.0.

Fawn Response. A survival strategy in which the child responds to perceived threat by becoming excessively compliant, people pleasing, and focused on keeping others happy. The fawn response can look like maturity or good behavior but is driven by the belief that safety depends on suppressing one's own needs and managing the emotions of others. See Chapters 3.0 and 8.0.

Felt Safety. The internal, body level experience of being safe enough to let your guard down. Felt safety is distinct from physical safety. A child can be physically safe in a loving home but not yet feel safe, because their nervous system is still running on templates formed during a dangerous earlier environment. Building felt safety is the foundational goal of trauma informed parenting. See Chapter 6.0.

HPA Axis. The hypothalamic pituitary adrenal axis, the body's central stress response system. When the amygdala detects threat, the HPA axis releases cortisol and adrenaline, preparing the body for fight or flight. In children with CPTSD, the HPA axis may be chronically activated (producing elevated cortisol) or blunted (producing insufficient cortisol), both of which have physical and emotional consequences. See Chapter 3.0.

Hyperarousal. A state of heightened physiological activation above the window of tolerance. The child is anxious, reactive, agitated, or aggressive. The sympathetic nervous system is engaged, preparing the body for action. See window of tolerance below and Chapter 3.0.

Hypoarousal. A state of reduced physiological activation below the window of tolerance. The child is shut down, numb, dissociated, or emotionally flat. The dorsal vagal system has engaged, conserving energy and reducing awareness. See window of tolerance below and Chapter 3.0.

Implicit Memory. Memories stored as fragments of sensation, emotion, and body response without a conscious narrative or time stamp. The child re-experiences the feeling, smell, sound, or bodily sensation of a past event without knowing that it is a memory. The body responds as though the danger is happening now. Implicit memories are the basis of most trauma triggers. See Chapter 3.0.

Manifestation Determination Review (MDR). A process required under the Individuals with Disabilities Education Act (IDEA) when a child with an IEP faces suspension or expulsion. The school team must determine whether the behavior was caused by or substantially related to the child's disability. If it was, the child cannot be removed from their placement without a plan to address the behavior through the IEP. See Chapter 13.0.

Negative Self Concept. A deep, persistent belief that one is bad, worthless, damaged, or fundamentally different from other people. In CPTSD, this belief forms during the developmental period when the child's sense of self is being constructed, and it is reinforced by the traumatic experiences. It is one of the three core features of CPTSD. See Chapter 2.0.

Neuroplasticity. The brain's ability to form new neural pathways in response to new experiences. Neuroplasticity means that the brain patterns formed by trauma can be reshaped through safe, attuned relationships and therapeutic support. It is the neurological basis for hope in CPTSD treatment. See Chapters 3.0 and 18.0.

PACE. An approach to building felt safety developed by Dan Hughes. PACE stands for Playfulness (bringing lightness and warmth), Acceptance (accepting the child's inner experience while setting limits on behavior), Curiosity (replacing judgment with wondering), and Empathy (sitting with the child's pain without trying to fix it). See Chapter 6.0.

Polyvagal Theory. A framework developed by Stephen Porges describing three states the nervous system operates in: ventral vagal (safe and social, where connection and learning happen), sympathetic activation (fight or flight, where the body mobilizes for action), and dorsal vagal (shutdown or collapse, where the body conserves energy and dissociation may occur). Understanding these states helps parents recognize what their child is experiencing in real time. See Chapter 3.0.

Rupture and Repair. The natural cycle in which a relationship experiences a disconnection (the caregiver misses a cue, loses their temper, or responds imperfectly) followed by a reconnection (the caregiver acknowledges the mistake and re-establishes the relationship). Repair is one of the most therapeutic things a parent can do, because it teaches the child that relationships can survive mistakes. See Chapter 7.0.

Secondary Traumatic Stress (STS). The impact of repeated exposure to another person's trauma. STS can produce symptoms that mirror PTSD: intrusive thoughts, hypervigilance, sleep disruption, emotional numbing, and a persistent sense of dread. It is well documented in professionals who work with trauma and is equally relevant for parents of traumatized children. See Chapter 16.0.

Sympathetic Activation. The fight or flight state in polyvagal theory. The body has mobilized for action: heart rate increases, muscles tense, and the child may become aggressive, restless, or attempt to flee. See polyvagal theory above and Chapter 3.0.

Trigger. Any stimulus that activates the trauma response. Triggers can be sensory (a sound, smell, texture), relational (a tone of voice, a facial expression), situational (transitions, new places), or temporal (anniversaries, certain times of day). Triggers activate implicit memory, causing the child's body to respond as though the original danger is present. See Chapters 3.0 and 8.0.

Ventral Vagal State. The safe and social state in polyvagal theory. The child feels calm, connected, and able to engage with others. Learning, play, and relationship building happen in this state. It is the state parents are working to help their child access more frequently and sustain for longer periods. See polyvagal theory above and Chapter 3.0.

Window of Tolerance. A concept introduced by Daniel Siegel describing the zone of arousal in which a person can function well. Inside the window, the child can think, feel, and respond. Above it, they are in hyperarousal. Below it, hypoarousal. For children with CPTSD, the window is narrow, meaning small provocations can push them out of it. The window can be widened over time through safe relationships, co-regulation, and therapy. See Chapter 3.0.

Appendix B: Printable Tools and Worksheets

The following tools are designed to be used in daily life. Print them, photocopy them, or recreate them in a notebook. They are most useful when completed regularly over time, because patterns become visible only through consistent tracking.

Trigger Mapping Worksheet

Use this worksheet each time your child has a significant behavioral reaction. Complete it as soon as possible after the event, when details are fresh. After one to two weeks of consistent tracking, review the entries and look for patterns.

Date and time: _________________

Location: _______________

What happened immediately before the reaction (the event, transition, interaction, or sensory input that preceded the behavior): _______________

What the behavior looked like (describe what the child did, not what you think it meant): _______________

Which nervous system state did this seem to reflect? (Check one)
( ) Fight (aggression, yelling, hitting, throwing) ( ) Flight (running, bolting, trying to escape) ( ) Freeze/Collapse (going blank, staring, unresponsive, limp) ( ) Fawn (sudden compliance, people pleasing, apologizing excessively)

What was happening in the environment? (Noise level, people present, changes to routine, sensory factors): _______________

How long did the reaction last? _______________

What helped the child return to baseline? _________________

What did not help or made it worse? ______________

Possible trigger (your best guess about what activated the response): ________________

Notes for your child's therapist: ______________

Behavior Translation Journal

This journal helps you practice interpreting your child's behavior through a trauma lens. Complete one entry per day, choosing the most significant behavioral moment. Over time, this practice rewires your own response patterns.

Date: ___________________

What the child did (the visible behavior): ___________________

What I think they were feeling (the emotion underneath the behavior): ___________________

What the behavior might have been trying to accomplish (the function): ___________________

What the child would say if they had the words:

____

How I responded: ___________________

How I wish I had responded (if different): ___________________

What I want to remember for next time: ___________________

Family Crisis Safety Plan

Complete this plan during a calm period. Post it in an accessible location. Make sure every adult in the household knows where it is and what it says. Review and update it every three months or after any significant change in your child's needs.

Emergency contacts: Child's therapist (name and phone): ________________ Child's psychiatrist (name and phone): ________________ Child's pediatrician (name and phone): ________________ Local crisis line: ________________ National crisis line: 988 (Suicide and Crisis Lifeline) Nearest emergency department (name and address): ________________

Child's current medications (name, dose, time):

    1. ____
    2. ____
    3. ____

De-escalation strategies that work for this child:

    1. ____
    2. ____
    3. ____

De-escalation strategies that do NOT work for this child (do not use these during crisis):

    1. ____
    2. ____

Safety plan for other family members during a crisis: Who takes the siblings to another room: ________________ Who stays with the child in crisis: ________________ Where siblings go if they need to leave the house: ________________

When to call for professional help: Call the therapist when: ________________ Call 988 or go to the emergency department when: ________________

Post-crisis plan: Who checks in with the child after they are regulated: ________________ Who checks in with siblings: ________________ Who debriefs with the other parent/caregiver: ________________

Therapist Screening Checklist

Use this checklist during your initial phone consultation with a potential therapist. Take notes on the responses. Trust your instincts about fit.

Therapist name: ___________________ Date of call: ___________________ Licensure type (LCSW, LPC, LMFT, PhD, PsyD): ___________________

( ) What is your training and experience with complex trauma in children? Notes: ___________________

( ) Are you familiar with CPTSD (ICD-11) and Developmental Trauma Disorder? Notes: ___________________

( ) Which evidence-based modalities do you use? (TF-CBT, ARC, EMDR, CPP, DBT, play therapy, somatic approaches) Notes: ___________________

( ) How do you approach the first phase of treatment? Notes:

____

( ) How do you involve caregivers in the treatment process? Notes: ___________________

( ) What does progress typically look like, and what is a realistic timeline? Notes: ___________________

( ) How do you handle crises between sessions? Notes:

____

( ) Do you coordinate with schools, psychiatrists, and other providers? Notes: ___________________

( ) What insurance do you accept, or do you provide superbills for out-of-network reimbursement? Notes: ___________________

Overall impression: _________________ Proceed with intake? ( )
Yes ( ) No ( ) Maybe, need more information

IEP/504 Accommodation Request Template

Adapt this template and send it (by email or certified mail) to your child's school principal and director of special education. Keep a copy for your records.

Date: ________________

To: [Principal name], [School name] CC: [Director of Special Education]

Re: Request for [IEP Evaluation under IDEA / Section 504 Plan] for [Child's name], [Grade], [Date of birth]

Dear [Principal name],

I am writing to formally request [an evaluation for an Individualized Education Program (IEP) under the Individuals with Disabilities Education Act / a Section 504 Plan under Section 504 of the Rehabilitation Act] for my child, [name].

[Child's name] has been diagnosed with [diagnosis, e.g., PTSD, anxiety disorder, adjustment disorder] which substantially affects their ability to [list specific functional impacts, such as: regulate emotions in the classroom, manage transitions between activities, sustain attention during instruction, interact appropriately with peers, tolerate sensory stimulation in common areas].

Specific concerns include: [list 3-5 observable behaviors or functional limitations the school has documented or that you have observed].

I am requesting that the school conduct a full evaluation to determine eligibility for [an IEP / a 504 Plan] and to identify appropriate accommodations and services. I understand the school has [your state's timeline, typically 60 calendar days] to complete this evaluation after consent is provided.

I have enclosed [or: I will provide upon request] documentation from [child's therapist/psychiatrist name], including a summary of functional limitations and recommended accommodations.

Please confirm receipt of this request in writing and provide the next steps in the evaluation process.

Thank you for your attention to this matter. I look forward to working collaboratively to support [child's name]'s educational success.

Sincerely, [Your name] [Your contact information]

Caregiver STS Self-Assessment

Rate each item from 0 (not at all) to 4 (very much) based on your experience over the past 30 days. This is not a diagnostic tool. It is a self-awareness check to help you recognize when you need additional support. Adapted from concepts in the Professional Quality of Life Scale (Stamm, 2010).

1. I have difficulty sleeping because of thoughts about my child's trauma history. (0 1 2 3 4)
2. I feel emotionally numb or disconnected from my own life. (0 1 2 3 4)
3. I am more irritable than usual, and small things set me off. (0 1 2 3 4)
4. I have intrusive thoughts or images related to what my child has experienced. (0 1 2 3 4)
5. I feel trapped in this caregiving situation with no way out. (0 1 2 3 4)
6. I have lost interest in activities that used to bring me enjoyment. (0 1 2 3 4)
7. I find it hard to concentrate or make decisions. (0 1 2 3 4)
8. I have withdrawn from friends, family, or my partner. (0 1 2 3 4)
9. I experience physical symptoms (headaches, stomach problems, fatigue) that I did not have before. (0 1 2 3 4)
10. I feel like I am going through the motions of caregiving without emotional connection. (0 1 2 3 4)

Scoring guide: 0 to 10: Low current impact. Continue monitoring. 11 to 25: Moderate impact. Consider increasing support (therapy, respite, support group). 26 to 40: High impact. Seek professional support promptly. You deserve care too. See Chapter 16.0.

Daily Regulation Check-In

Use this brief check-in once per day (morning or evening) to track your own nervous system state. Over time, patterns will emerge that help you anticipate your own needs.

Date: ___________________

My energy level today (1 = depleted, 5 = resourced): ____

My patience level today (1 = very low, 5 = steady): ____

My emotional state today (circle all that apply): Calm / Anxious / Irritable / Sad / Numb / Overwhelmed / Hopeful / Angry / Connected / Disconnected

One thing that helped me today: ___________________

One thing that was hard today: ________________

What I need tomorrow: ________________

Appendix C: Recommended Reading and Resources

The following resources are organized by category and annotated with brief descriptions to help you identify which ones are most relevant to your current needs.

Books for Parents and Caregivers

The Body Keeps the Score by Bessel van der Kolk (2014). The most widely read book on trauma and the body. Dense but essential. Read Part Five first if you want practical applications before the neuroscience. Not specific to children, but foundational.

The Connected Child by Karyn Purvis, David Cross, and Wendy Sunshine (2013). Written specifically for adoptive and foster parents. Practical, accessible, and grounded in the Trust-Based Relational Intervention (TBRI) model. One of the best starting points for parents new to trauma informed parenting.

The Whole-Brain Child by Daniel Siegel and Tina Payne Bryson (2011). Explains brain development in plain language with specific strategies for common parenting challenges. Not trauma specific, but highly applicable. The "name it to tame it" framework is immediately usable.

Brain-Based Parenting by Daniel Hughes and Jonathan Baylin (2012). A deeper look at the neuroscience of caregiving. Explains why parenting a traumatized child changes the parent's brain, and what to do about it. More clinical than some entries on this list, but invaluable.

Attachment-Focused Parenting by Daniel Hughes (2009). A practical guide to implementing PACE (Playfulness, Acceptance,

Curiosity, Empathy) in daily parenting. Particularly relevant to Chapters 6.0 and 7.0 of this book.

Trauma and Recovery by Judith Herman (2015, revised edition). The foundational text on complex trauma. Originally written about adult survivors, but the framework (phase-based treatment, understanding the impact of relational trauma) applies directly to understanding your child.

The Boy Who Was Raised as a Dog by Bruce Perry and Maia Szalavitz (2006). Case studies of children Perry treated, written in accessible narrative form. Powerful for understanding how different types of early adversity produce different patterns of behavior and development.

Complex PTSD: From Surviving to Thriving by Pete Walker (2013). Written for adult survivors, but many parents of children with CPTSD find it illuminating for understanding their child's inner experience, and for understanding their own.

Beyond Consequences, Logic, and Control by Heather Forbes and Bryan Post (2009). A practical guide to responding to difficult behavior through a trauma lens. Short chapters organized around specific behavioral challenges.

Books for Children and Teens

A Terrible Thing Happened by Margaret Holmes, illustrated by Cary Pillo (2000). A picture book for young children (ages 4 to 8) about a raccoon who witnessed something terrible and learns to talk about his feelings with a counselor. Gentle and accessible.

The Invisible String by Patrice Karst (2018). A picture book about the invisible connection between people who love each other, even when they are apart. Useful for children dealing with separation, placement changes, or attachment anxiety.

Trauma Is Really Strange by Steve Haines, illustrated by Sophie Standing (2016). A short graphic book explaining trauma and the body in simple, visual terms. Appropriate for older children and teenagers.

What Happened to You? by Oprah Winfrey and Bruce Perry (2021). Accessible for older teens. Reframes "What's wrong with you?" as "What happened to you?" and explains trauma's impact on the brain and body.

Organizations and Crisis Hotlines

National Child Traumatic Stress Network (NCTSN): nctsn.org. The leading resource for information about childhood trauma, evidence-based treatments, and provider directories. Their "Resources for Families" section is written specifically for parents.

988 Suicide and Crisis Lifeline: Call or text 988 (United States). Available 24 hours a day, 7 days a week. Provides free, confidential support for people in distress and for caregivers concerned about a loved one.

Crisis Text Line: Text HOME to 741741 (United States). Free, confidential crisis counseling via text message. Available 24/7.

ARCH National Respite Network: archrespite.org. Helps families locate respite care services in their state. Includes information about respite funding sources.

North American Council on Adoptable Children (NACAC): nacac.org. Support groups, educational resources, and advocacy for adoptive families.

National Alliance for Mental Illness (NAMI): nami.org. Family support groups, educational programs, and a helpline (1-800-950-NAMI) for families navigating mental health challenges.

Attachment and Trauma Network (ATN): attachmenttraumanetwork.org. Specifically serves families raising children with trauma and attachment challenges. Offers online support groups and educational resources.

Child Welfare Information Gateway: childwelfare.gov. Information on foster care, adoption, child welfare systems, and services for families. Published by the U.S. Department of Health and Human Services.

Therapeutic Provider Directories

Psychology Today Therapist Finder (psychologytoday.com/us/therapists): Filter by "trauma," your child's age, insurance, and location.

EMDR International Association (emdria.org/find-an-emdr-therapist): Directory of EMDR-trained and certified therapists.

National Child Traumatic Stress Network (nctsn.org): Locate NCTSN member sites and affiliated providers in your area.

TF-CBT Therapist Certification Program (tfcbt.org): Information about TF-CBT trained therapists and training resources.

Association for Play Therapy (a4pt.org): Directory of registered play therapists.

Appendix D: Letter to Your Child's Teacher

The following template is designed to be photocopied, adapted, and given to your child's teacher at the beginning of the school year or whenever a new teacher enters your child's life. It communicates what your child needs without disclosing the specific details of their trauma history. Adapt the language to fit your child's age and presentation.

Dear [Teacher's name],

Thank you for having [child's name] in your classroom this year. I wanted to share some information that I hope will help you understand and support [him/her/them] as effectively as possible.

[Child's name] has experienced significant early life adversity that has affected the way [his/her/their] brain processes stress, manages emotions, and responds to the environment. This is not a discipline issue. It is a neurological reality. [He/She/They] is working with a therapist and making progress, and your classroom is an important part of that progress.

What you may notice:

[Child's name] may have difficulty with transitions between activities, especially when they are unexpected. [He/She/They] may react to changes in routine with anxiety, withdrawal, or agitation that seems out of proportion to the change.

[He/She/They] may have difficulty sustaining attention, not because of disinterest, but because [his/her/their] nervous system is working hard to feel safe in the environment. Hypervigilance (scanning for exits, watching adult facial expressions, startling at sudden sounds) may look like inattention.

[He/She/They] may occasionally "shut down" or go blank. This is called dissociation, and it is a stress response, not defiance or daydreaming. It passes more quickly with gentle, sensory-based redirection (saying their name calmly, asking if they can feel their feet on the floor) than with raised voices or physical touch.

[He/She/They] may have strong emotional reactions to situations that seem minor. These reactions are driven by a sensitive alarm system in the brain, not by willfulness or manipulation.

What helps:

- Advance notice before transitions or changes to routine ("In five minutes, we are going to switch to math.")
- A designated safe person [child's name] can go to when feeling overwhelmed
- A safe space in or near the classroom where [he/she/they] can regulate without it being framed as punishment
- Low, calm vocal tone when giving directions, especially during moments of escalation
- Avoiding public correction or consequences delivered in front of peers
- Permission to use sensory supports (fidget tools, noise-canceling headphones, movement breaks)
- Brief check-ins at the beginning and end of the day with a trusted adult

What does not help:

- Raised voices, even when directed at other students (this can activate [child's name]'s stress response)
- Surprise schedule changes without warning
- Being singled out or called on unexpectedly in front of the class

- Loss of recess as a consequence (movement helps regulate the nervous system)
- Being sent to sit alone as a disciplinary measure (isolation can feel like abandonment to a child with this history)

What I am not asking you to do:

I am not asking you to treat [child's name] differently from every other student. I am asking you to understand that [his/her/their] brain responds to stress differently, and that small environmental adjustments can make the difference between a day of learning and a day of crisis.

I am not sharing the details of [child's name]'s history, because that information belongs to [him/her/them]. What I am sharing is what you need to know to support [him/her/them] in your classroom.

I would welcome the chance to talk with you further, and I am happy to connect you with [child's name]'s therapist (with your agreement) for additional guidance.

Thank you for your care and attention. Your classroom matters more than you know to a child who is learning that the world can be a safe place.

Sincerely, [Your name] [Your contact information]

Appendix E: Higher Levels of Care

There may come a time when outpatient therapy, school accommodations, and your best parenting efforts are not enough. When your child's safety is at persistent risk. When the family system is in crisis. When you have tried everything this book recommends and the situation continues to deteriorate. This appendix is for that moment.

Seeking a higher level of care is not failure. It is a recognition that your child's needs have exceeded what can be met in the current setting, and that a more intensive environment may be what they need to stabilize before returning home.

Understanding the Levels

Mental health care exists on a continuum of intensity. From least to most intensive, the levels most relevant to children with CPTSD are the following.

Outpatient therapy is what most of this book has described: weekly or biweekly sessions with a therapist, supplemented by psychiatric care if needed. This is appropriate for children who are stable enough to function in their daily environment with support.

Intensive outpatient programs (IOP) provide structured therapeutic programming for several hours per day, several days per week, while the child continues to live at home. IOPs typically include group therapy, individual therapy, family sessions, and skill building. They are a step up from weekly outpatient and can be effective when a child needs more support than one session per week provides but does not require 24 hour care.

Partial hospitalization programs (PHP), sometimes called day treatment, provide full day therapeutic programming (typically five to six hours) while the child returns home each evening. PHPs offer the intensity of inpatient care without the overnight separation. They are appropriate for children who are in acute distress but whose safety can be maintained at home overnight.

Residential treatment centers (RTC) provide 24 hour care in a structured therapeutic environment. The child lives at the facility and participates in a daily program that includes therapy, education, and life skills. Residential stays typically last several months, though duration varies. RTCs are appropriate when the child's behavior poses a persistent safety risk that cannot be managed at home, or when the child needs an extended period of stabilization that outpatient and day treatment have not been able to provide.

Inpatient psychiatric hospitalization is the most intensive and most restrictive level. It is appropriate for acute psychiatric emergencies: active suicidal behavior, severe self harm, psychotic episodes, or dangerous aggression that poses immediate risk. Inpatient stays are typically short (days to weeks) and are designed to stabilize the crisis, not to provide long term treatment.

Evaluating Programs for Trauma Competence

Not all residential programs or intensive treatment settings are equipped to work with CPTSD. Some use behavioral modification approaches (point systems, privilege levels, confrontational groups) that are counterproductive for traumatized children. Before placing your child in any program, ask the following questions.

What is your treatment philosophy? (You are looking for language about trauma informed care, relational approaches, and phase-based treatment. Programs that emphasize compliance,

earned privileges, and behavioral control as their primary
framework may not be appropriate.)

What evidence-based modalities do your therapists use? (Look
for TF-CBT, ARC, EMDR, DBT, somatic approaches, and play
therapy. Ask about staff training and supervision.)

How do you handle behavioral crises? (You are looking for de-
escalation protocols, not physical restraint as a first response. Ask
specifically about the use of seclusion and restraint, and request
the facility's restraint data.)

How are families involved in treatment? (A program that
excludes families or limits contact to brief phone calls may
undermine the attachment work you have been building. Look for
programs that include regular family therapy, parent education,
and a clear plan for reintegration.)

What is your approach to medication? (Ask who prescribes, how
often the child is seen, and whether medication changes are
communicated to parents in advance.)

What is your staff-to-child ratio, and what training do direct care
staff receive? (The people who spend the most time with your
child are often the least clinically trained. Ask about trauma
training for all staff, not just therapists.)

Can I visit the facility before making a decision? (Any program
that discourages parent visits should raise concerns.)

Maintaining Connection During Placement

If your child enters a residential or inpatient setting, maintaining
your connection with them is critical. The child's nervous system
already carries the template that adults leave when things get
hard. A residential placement can feel, to the child, like another
in a long line of abandonments, even when it is the most loving
choice you could make.

Stay involved. Attend every family session. Make every scheduled phone call. Write letters. Send drawings. Ask the treatment team what you can do from home to reinforce the work they are doing on site.

When the child says, "You sent me away," (and they may), respond honestly: "I sent you to a place where you could get more help than I could give you at home. I did not leave. I am here. I am coming to visit. And I am working to bring you home."

Consider Oswin (name changed), the 14 year old from Chapter 5.0. When he was placed in a therapeutic day program, his foster mother was initially relieved and then devastated by guilt. His therapist reframed the decision: "You are not giving up on him. You are getting him what he needs in the environment that can provide it. And you are still his person. That hasn't changed." She visited every Friday, and Oswin, who had initially refused to speak to her, began greeting her at the door by the second month.

Transition Planning

The transition home from a higher level of care is as important as the placement itself. Without a clear plan, the gains made during treatment can erode quickly when the child returns to the environment where the difficulties originated.

A good transition plan includes the following. A step-down schedule (for example, transitioning from residential to day treatment to intensive outpatient before returning to standard outpatient care). Updated accommodations and supports at school, communicated in advance of the child's return. Continued therapy with a provider who has received a thorough handoff from the treatment facility. A family session (or series of sessions) focused specifically on reintegration: rebuilding routines, resetting expectations, and processing the separation for both the child and the family. An updated safety plan that reflects what was learned during treatment about the child's triggers, effective interventions, and warning signs of deterioration.

Request that the treatment facility provide a written discharge summary and aftercare recommendations. Bring these to your child's outpatient team, school, and prescriber. The information gathered during intensive treatment is valuable and should not be lost in the transition.

You Are Still the Constant

Whatever level of care your child needs, you remain the constant in their life. Programs end. Therapists change. Caseworkers rotate. But you are the person who was there before the placement and will be there after. Your presence, your persistence, and your willingness to make the hard decisions (including the decision to seek a higher level of care when needed) are the thread that runs through your child's story.

This is not an easy part of the story. But it is not the end of it.

References

- American Academy of Child and Adolescent Psychiatry. (2009). Practice parameter on the use of psychotropic medication in children and adolescents. *Journal of the American Academy of Child and Adolescent Psychiatry, 48*(9), 961–973.
- American Psychiatric Association. (2013). *Diagnostic and statistical manual of mental disorders* (5th ed.). American Psychiatric Publishing.
- ARCH National Respite Network. (n.d.). *Find respite and crisis care services in your state.* ARCH National Respite Network.
- Baylin, J., & Hughes, D. A. (2016). *The neurobiology of attachment-focused therapy: Enhancing connection and trust in the treatment of children and adolescents.* W. W. Norton.
- Beacon House. (2020). *The iceberg of behaviour.* Beacon House Therapeutic Services and Trauma Team.
- Blaustein, M. E., & Kinniburgh, K. M. (2018). *Treating traumatic stress in children and adolescents: How to foster resilience through attachment, self-regulation, and competency* (2nd ed.). Guilford Press.
- Bombèr, L. M. (2007). *Inside I'm hurting: Practical strategies for supporting children with attachment difficulties in schools.* Worth Publishing.
- Chaffin, M., Hanson, R., Saunders, B. E., Nichols, T., Barnett, D., Zeanah, C., Berliner, L., Egeland, B., Newman, E., Lyon, T., Letourneau, E., & Miller-Perrin, C. (2006). Report of the APSAC Task Force on attachment therapy, reactive attachment disorder, and attachment problems. *Child Maltreatment, 11*(1), 76–89.
- Child Welfare Information Gateway. (2019). *Adoption assistance for children adopted from foster care.* U.S. Department of Health and Human Services,

Administration for Children and Families, Children's Bureau.

- Cloitre, M., Courtois, C. A., Charuvastra, A., Carapezza, R., Stolbach, B. C., & Green, B. L. (2011). Treatment of complex PTSD: Results of the ISTSS expert clinician survey on best practices. *Journal of Traumatic Stress, 24*(6), 615–627.
- Cloitre, M., Garvert, D. W., Brewin, C. R., Bryant, R. A., & Maercker, A. (2013). Evidence for proposed ICD-11 PTSD and complex PTSD: A latent profile analysis. *European Journal of Psychotraumatology, 4*(1), 20706.
- Cohen, J. A., Mannarino, A. P., & Deblinger, E. (2017). *Treating trauma and traumatic grief in children and adolescents* (2nd ed.). Guilford Press.
- Cole, S. F., O'Brien, J. G., Gadd, M. G., Ristuccia, J., Wallace, D. L., & Gregory, M. (2005). *Helping traumatized children learn: Supportive school environments for children traumatized by family violence.* Massachusetts Advocates for Children.
- Cook, A., Spinazzola, J., Ford, J., Lanktree, C., Blaustein, M., Cloitre, M., DeRosa, R., Hubbard, R., Liautaud, J., Olafson, E., Kagan, R., Mallah, K., & van der Kolk, B. (2005). Complex trauma in children and adolescents. *Psychiatric Annals, 35*(5), 390–398.
- Feinberg, M. E., Solmeyer, A. R., & McHale, S. M. (2012). The third rail of family systems: Sibling relationships, mental and behavioral health, and preventive intervention in childhood and adolescence. *Clinical Child and Family Psychology Review, 15*(1), 43–57.
- Figley, C. R. (2002). Compassion fatigue: Psychotherapists' chronic lack of self-care. *Journal of Clinical Psychology, 58*(11), 1433–1441.
- Ford, J. D., & Courtois, C. A. (2020). *Treating complex traumatic stress disorders in adults* (2nd ed.). Guilford Press.

- Gunnar, M. R., & Quevedo, K. (2007). The neurobiology of stress and development. *Annual Review of Psychology, 58*, 145–173.
- Hartley, S. L., Barker, E. T., Seltzer, M. M., Floyd, F., Greenberg, J., Orsmond, G., & Bolt, D. (2010). The relative risk and timing of divorce in families of children with an autism spectrum disorder. *Journal of Family Psychology, 24*(4), 449–457.
- Herman, J. L. (2015). *Trauma and recovery: The aftermath of violence from domestic abuse to political terror* (Rev. ed.). Basic Books.
- Hughes, D. A. (2009). *Attachment-focused parenting: Effective strategies to care for children.* W. W. Norton.
- Hughes, D. A., & Baylin, J. (2012). *Brain-based parenting: The neuroscience of caregiving for healthy attachment.* W. W. Norton.
- Individuals with Disabilities Education Act, 20 U.S.C. § 1400 (2004).
- Kerns, C. M., Newschaffer, C. J., & Berkowitz, S. J. (2015). Traumatic childhood events and autism spectrum disorder. *Journal of Autism and Developmental Disorders, 45*(11), 3475–3486.
- Landreth, G. L. (2012). *Play therapy: The art of the relationship* (3rd ed.). Routledge.
- LeDoux, J. E. (2015). *Anxious: Using the brain to understand and treat fear and anxiety.* Viking.
- Levine, P. A., & Kline, M. (2007). *Trauma through a child's eyes: Awakening the ordinary miracle of healing.* North Atlantic Books.
- Lieberman, A. F., & Van Horn, P. (2005). *Don't hit my mommy! A manual for child-parent psychotherapy with young children exposed to violence and other trauma.* Zero to Three.
- Miller, A. L., Rathus, J. H., & Linehan, M. M. (2007). *Dialectical behavior therapy with suicidal adolescents.* Guilford Press.

- National Child Traumatic Stress Network. (n.d.). *Empirically supported treatments and promising practices.* National Child Traumatic Stress Network.
- National Child Traumatic Stress Network. (n.d.). *Resources for families and caregivers.* National Child Traumatic Stress Network.
- National Child Traumatic Stress Network. (2018). *Complex trauma: Facts for caregivers.* National Child Traumatic Stress Network.
- Perry, B. D., & Szalavitz, M. (2006). *The boy who was raised as a dog: And other stories from a child psychiatrist's notebook.* Basic Books.
- Porges, S. W. (2011). *The polyvagal theory: Neurophysiological foundations of emotions, attachment, communication, and self-regulation.* W. W. Norton.
- Purvis, K. B., Cross, D. R., & Sunshine, W. L. (2013). *The connected child: Bring hope and healing to your adoptive family.* McGraw-Hill.
- Rutter, M., Beckett, C., Castle, J., Colvert, E., Kreppner, J., Mehta, M., Stevens, S., & Sonuga-Barke, E. (2007). Effects of profound early institutional deprivation: An overview of findings from a UK longitudinal study of Romanian adoptees. *European Journal of Developmental Psychology, 4*(3), 332–350.
- Shapiro, F. (2018). *Eye movement desensitization and reprocessing (EMDR) therapy: Basic principles, protocols, and procedures* (3rd ed.). Guilford Press.
- Siegel, D. J. (2012). *The developing mind: How relationships and the brain interact to shape who we are* (2nd ed.). Guilford Press.
- Siegel, D. J. (2014). *Brainstorm: The power and purpose of the teenage brain.* Tarcher/Penguin.
- Siegel, D. J., & Bryson, T. P. (2011). *The whole-brain child: 12 revolutionary strategies to nurture your child's developing mind.* Delacorte Press.
- Spinazzola, J., van der Kolk, B., & Ford, J. D. (2018). When nowhere is safe: Interpersonal trauma and attachment adversity as antecedents of posttraumatic

stress disorder and developmental trauma disorder. *Journal of Traumatic Stress, 31*(5), 631–642.

- Stamm, B. H. (2010). *The concise ProQOL manual* (2nd ed.). ProQOL.org.
- Substance Abuse and Mental Health Services Administration. (2014). *SAMHSA's concept of trauma and guidance for a trauma-informed approach.* U.S. Department of Health and Human Services.
- Szymanski, K., Sapanski, L., & Conway, F. (2011). Trauma and ADHD: Association or diagnostic confusion? A clinical perspective. *Journal of Infant, Child, and Adolescent Psychotherapy, 10*(1), 51–59.
- van der Kolk, B. A. (2005). Developmental trauma disorder: Toward a rational diagnosis for children with complex trauma histories. *Psychiatric Annals, 35*(5), 401–408.
- van der Kolk, B. A. (2014). *The body keeps the score: Brain, mind, and body in the healing of trauma.* Viking.
- van der Kolk, B. A., Hodgdon, H., Gapen, M., Musicaro, R., Suvak, M. K., Hamlin, E., & Spinazzola, J. (2016). A randomized controlled study of neurofeedback for chronic PTSD. *PLOS ONE, 11*(12), e0166752.
- Walker, P. (2013). *Complex PTSD: From surviving to thriving.* Azure Coyote Publishing.
- Warner, E., Koomar, J., Lary, B., & Cook, A. (2013). Can the body change the score? Application of sensory modulation principles in the treatment of traumatized adolescents in residential settings. *Journal of Family Violence, 28*(7), 729–738.
- Winnicott, D. W. (1971). *Playing and reality.* Tavistock Publications.
- World Health Organization. (2018). *International classification of diseases for mortality and morbidity statistics* (11th rev.). World Health Organization.
- Wright, P. W. D., & Wright, P. D. (2007). *Wrightslaw: From emotions to advocacy* (2nd ed.). Harbor House Law Press.